# Twinning It!

**murdoch books**

Sydney | London

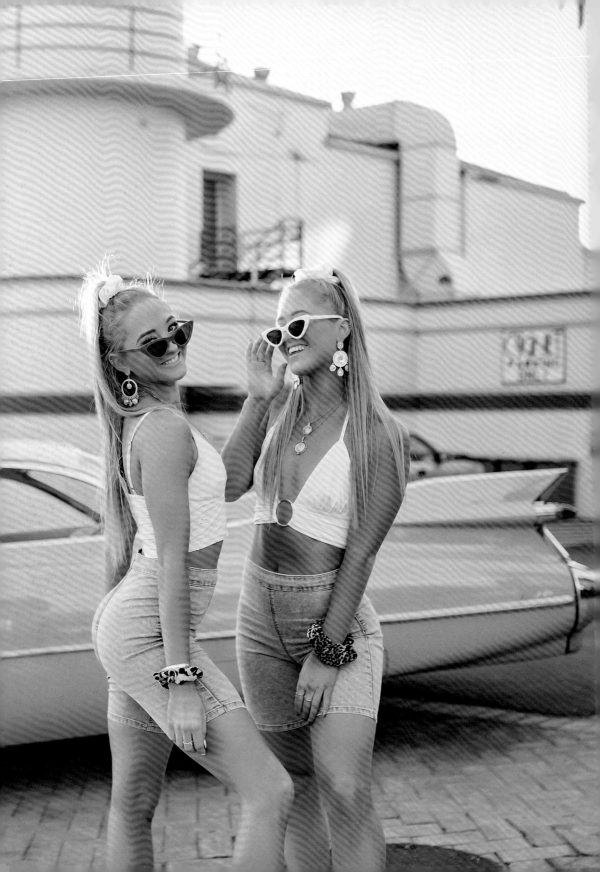

# Twinning It!

Dance, acro, friendship, YouTube & living life to the fullest

## SAM and TEAGAN RYBKA

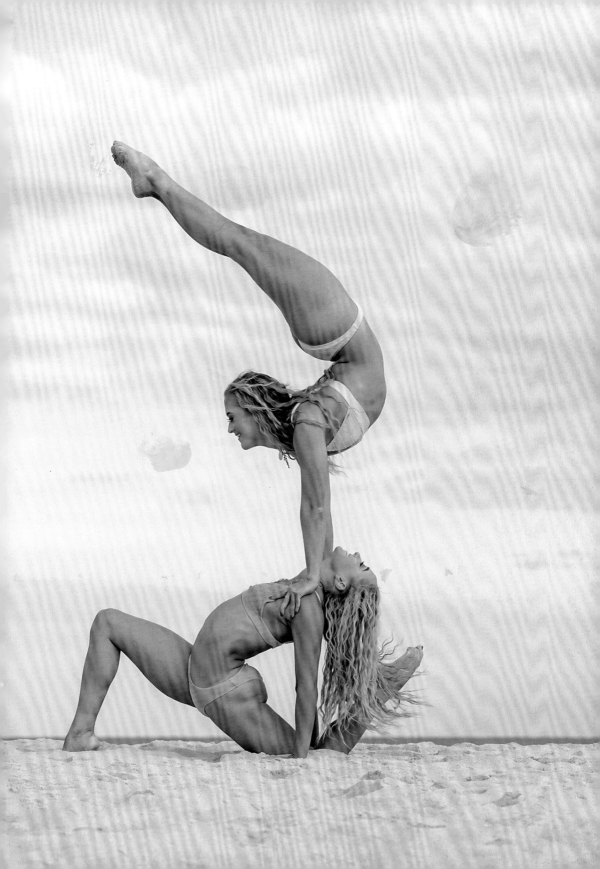

Teagan
xo

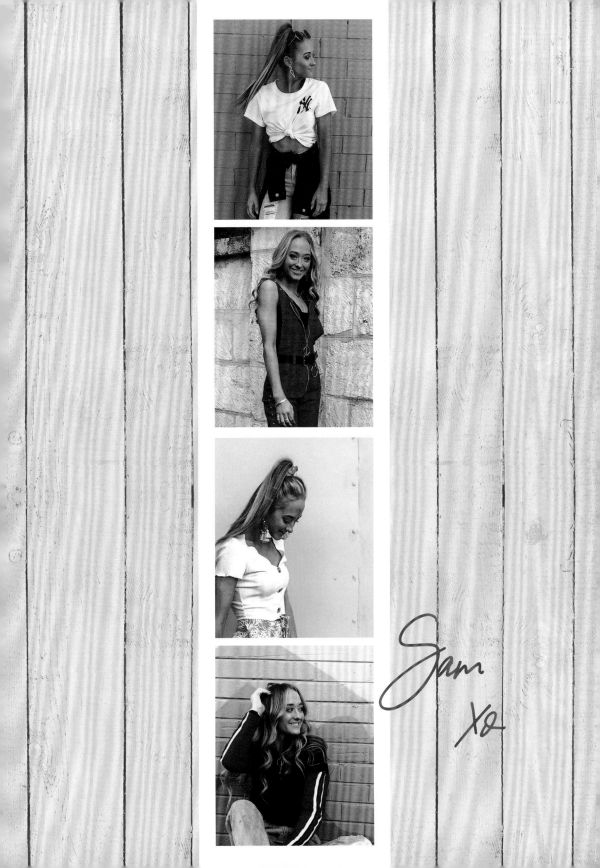

Sam
xo

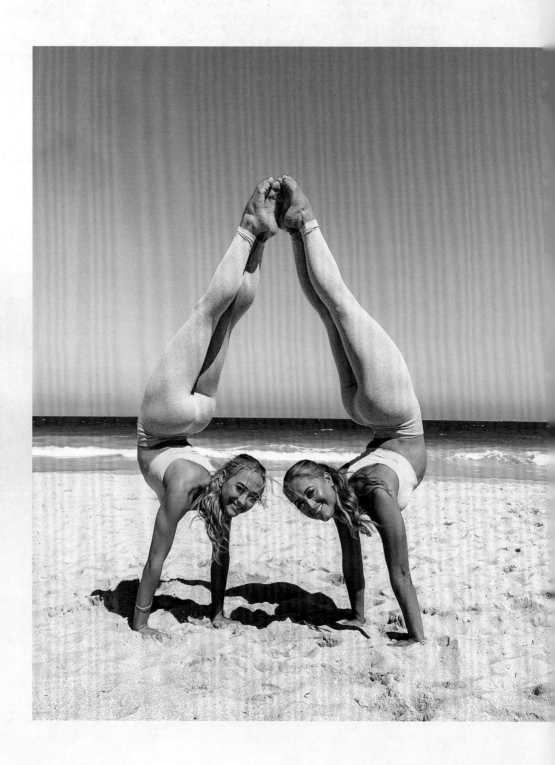

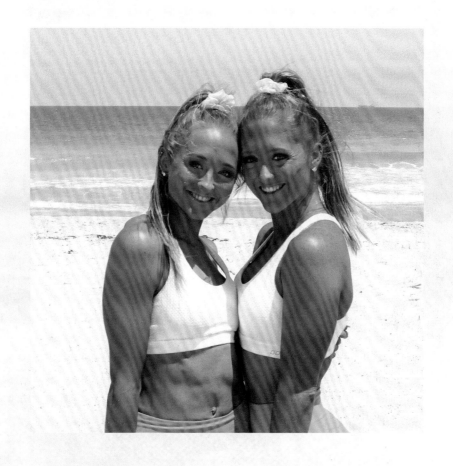

Beach days = best days

We'd like to dedicate this book
to the three Fs:
our family, friends and fans.
We wouldn't be where we are today
without all your love and support
on this crazy roller-coaster
of a ride called life.
Love,

*Teagan*
xo

*Sam*
xo

# contents

# Hey guys!

I'm Teagan.
I'm Sam.
And we are the Rybka twins.
Welcome to
our ~~channel~~ … **BOOK!**

We can't believe that we've written a book, and we can't believe
that you're reading it. (Thank you so much for picking it up!) It never
crossed our minds that we'd be able to tell our story this way one day,
but then, we didn't set out to do half of the things people know us for.

When we think about the things we've been able to do, it's insane.
We've met people we admire and had the opportunity to perform
for them; we've travelled all over the world and made awesome new
friends; and we've been able to share our love of dance and acro
with millions of people—not just on TV but on social media, too.
Each of these things has been a big deal to us.

And best of all, we've done this TOGETHER! Even though we can
do things on our own, we are better, and happier, together—being
a team is all we've ever known. We feel so lucky to have each other.
Certain things in our lives have been difficult, and we still have
our challenges, as anybody does, but we know that our lives have
probably been easier because we have had each other. Family and
friends make our world go around!

It's still hard for us to believe that our YouTube channel has millions
of subscribers who come back week after week to check in with what
we're doing and support us. Because of them, we've been able to take
the thing we love the most and turn it into our full-time jobs.

People all around the world send us messages telling us that
watching our videos makes them feel happier. They'll comment

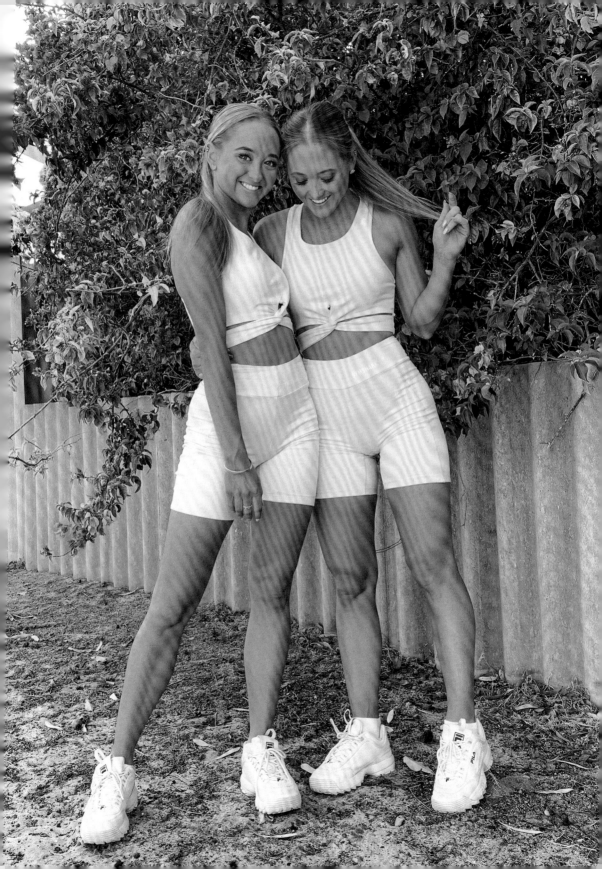

about how we are always smiling. When we film challenges where we compete against each other, we'll often get an influx of messages commenting on how good we are about losing to each other. But to us, it's so natural to be happy for the winner. We love creating the space in our community for that attitude—we should all be in this together. Real queens fix each other's crowns!

It's so crazy to us that we have this effect on people. Being able to make someone smile that day, or hearing people say that we inspire them, really motivates us. And we hope that our book can be another thing that adds positivity to your life. We hope that sharing our stories helps you understand that if you work hard and set goals, there are no limits to what you can achieve.

You never know when *something you say or do* will help someone, so we try to be as positive as we can, and to *make the most of everything.*

• • •

'In a world where you can be anything, be kind.' We see this quote from time to time, and while we aren't sure who said it first, we love it. It's such great advice. Unfortunately, we live in a world that can be quite negative, and we believe that any bit of positivity you put out there can help. You never know when something you say or do will help someone, so we try to be as positive as we can, and to make the most of everything. Usually we do this through YouTube, but now we get to do this in a book, too! We very much believe that you should try to be kind to everyone, because a little bit of kindness goes a long way.

# Where is dance going to lead?

When we were kids, dancing and acro were just these fun activities we did; they were the hobbies that we loved. But, as we got older and became more serious about competing and improving as dancers, we were often asked, 'So, what are going to do with your life?' or 'Where is dancing going to take you?'.

We didn't know! All we were sure of was that we loved dancing; it was all we thought about, and all we ever wanted to do. Perhaps people thought the hours we were spending dancing and competing were going to be wasted; perhaps they didn't see how we'd ever be able to do anything practical with dancing in Perth. Lots of people believe that you have to move to Sydney, or even to the United States, if you want to find work in dance. But we love living in Perth and are so grateful that we get to do what we love from home and can travel whenever we need to.

Even though we weren't sure exactly where dancing would lead, we kept going. And now, we get to dance all over the world, and we have opportunities we never dreamed of. So, when people ask us what we're going to do with dancing, we tell them we're already doing it! We're making a living, and we get to come home to our family at the end of the day. Everyone has to work, but not everyone gets to do the thing they love the most for a living. We feel so lucky that this thing we started doing for fun, that we love so much, has transitioned into our job.

Dancing has shaped us in so many ways and means so much to us. It meant a lot to our Mum in her life, too. Mum grew up in quite a poor family, and when she was little, her mother did everything she could to make sure her daughters could do dancing. She'd wanted to do it and couldn't, so she gave them that opportunity.

This had a big effect on Mum—those dance classes made her feel important. Dancing made her feel as if she belonged. It gave her goals to achieve and a sense of self-esteem, and she wanted to share that with us, and see if we'd love it, too. We did.

When we were in school, we were known as 'those acro twins'. Kids would say things like, 'They can do flips and stuff, and they're really flexible!' It was always a conversation starter, and it made us feel special. Not everyone feels they 'fit in' at school, but fitting in wasn't even on our minds. There wasn't room for it! We were always thinking about dancing, looking ahead to the next performance or competition, and too busy training to worry about whether we were in the 'right' group.

## Find that thing

We feel so lucky to have had the experiences we did growing up. It's important to find self-worth in something in life, but some kids aren't given the opportunity to find things they are good at. For whatever reason, they might never get a chance to try different sports or hobbies and get a feel for what they like or find out where their natural talents lie. Then suddenly, when they're in Year 10, adults start asking them what they want to do for a career, and they're stumped.

When we were asked this question, we knew we wanted careers that were tied to dance in some way, perhaps as a dance teacher or a performer. But if you never find something you really care about, it's hard to pick a job out of the air and say that's what you want to do for the rest of your life.

When we were little, Mum and Dad firmly believed that all the kids in our family should have interests outside of school. It didn't matter what it was, we just had to choose something.

It was important to them that we had dreams, and that we learned how to set goals and achieve them. The way they saw it, not every kid loves school, but if you have a hobby that you enjoy, then setting goals will come naturally from that. You'll want to improve and to achieve the next milestone—not because you have to, but because you love it.

When it comes to finding a hobby, there's no pressure! Try something, and if you don't like it, move to the next option until you find something that fits. (Just make sure you give it a proper chance first.) This way, even if you're not happy at school, you still have this thing you love to look forward to and to grow from.

When our brothers were young (that's right, we have brothers!), they each had the goal of being on a football grand-final team, and they were always kicking the football and working towards that. And each one of them achieved that goal. Now that they're older, camping and fishing is their outlet, and it's what they turn to.

## Learning how to come back *stronger* from *tough lessons* sets you up well in life.

• • •

We think kids can learn so much from doing something they care about, be it a sport such as footy or cricket, or dance. You learn about yourself and learn so many life lessons along the way.

Caring about a hobby, taking it seriously and working hard at it teaches you how to be a good sport. You're going to lose sometimes, or have things go wrong, but part of being a good competitor or participant is accepting that and moving on. Learning how to come back stronger from those tough lessons sets you up well in other areas of your life.

Renowned New York dance photographer Jordan Matter took this shot of us. He's amazing!

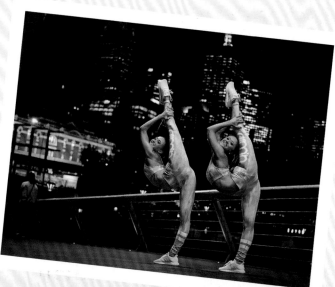

# When it came to hobbies, we didn't just dance

Most people think that all we've ever done in our lives is dance, but for two years during high school—Year 11 and Year 12—we also played netball, and absolutely loved it.

As part of the pathway-to-university subjects we did while still at high school, we had to join a team outside of school. Our hectic dance schedules made it almost impossible to find something we could do regularly, but then we found a netball team that played every Saturday at 8 am. (Argh! Early mornings aren't our favourite things.) Despite the early wake-up, we were happy about joining this team because we've always loved anything active, and we grew up with friends who were netballers; to be able to play ourselves was pretty cool.

Because everyone's schedules were jam-packed, we were never able to train with our team. This isn't good, and we aren't promoting doing that. If you're part of a team, you should definitely try to make it to all the training sessions. But even though we never trained together, we found we worked well together. We were all strangers at the start of the season but became close by the end of it. Because of that, we played well as a team—so well that we even won the grand final! This just proves that if you've got the right team or the right friends, you can conquer so much together.

We loved this experience because it was different to dancing— being part of a team and working together to try to win. Having that experience from a different perspective was so good.

We also took swimming lessons. When we were growing up, Mum wanted all of us kids to be strong swimmers, not only because we had a pool at home, but also because she wanted us to be able to help other people if we needed to. We took the regular swimming classes that everyone must do at school, but then every Christmas holiday, Mum would make us get up really early to go to lessons.

We still remember the feeling of jumping into a cold pool in the morning—that bit was not fun! We did this every summer for quite a few years until we got our Bronze Medallion (the level of swimming you need if you want to be a lifesaver).

## Dance is life!

Dancing has added so much to our lives. It hasn't just taught us movement and given us a love of music; it also taught us discipline and how to work in a team environment. It gives you a sense of self-worth and confidence (these are big ones!). Dance is also great for teaching you how to be dedicated, because if you aren't dedicated, you won't improve.

It's hard to put into words exactly why we love it as much as we do—it has just always felt so good to us to be able to express ourselves in different ways, especially to music. To have something we're good at and can be proud of is such a good feeling!

All the friendships and the memories we created through dancing are so special to us—it's like another world. And it makes us feel as if we belong. We feel like we've accomplished things in that world, whether they're small things, such as nailing a trick or complicated choreography, or big things, like winning competitions. Performing in front of people is the best feeling ever. And although dancing is hard work, it's still a lot of fun—and we're people who love fun!

So many kids have anxiety these days, and when we talked about anxiety briefly in a video once, we had a lot of people reach out and say they appreciated it so much.

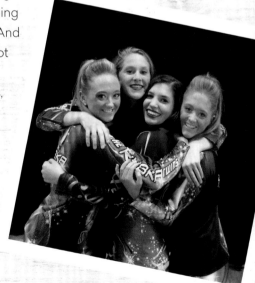

With Haley Huelsman and Ashtin Roth on the Edge of Dreams Tour.

Growing up, there were a few times we felt so nervous that we wouldn't want to get on stage, but we'd make ourselves do it, and this made us realise that we could do something, if we put our minds to it. That attitude started translating across to other areas of our life, such as school. We learned that running away isn't the answer, and that things usually aren't as bad you might imagine.

Nerves are an uncomfortable feeling, but when you're young, it's important to learn that they're a normal part of life—they usually come when something is important to you.

We like to help the kids we teach face these challenges and get over their fear, because if someone always has the option not to do something, they'll grow up without facing their fears and realising that they do have what it takes to get past them. Remember, even adults get anxious about certain things. Everybody gets nervous, but it feels so good to face your fears and accomplish something you were worried about.

We do understand that nerves and anxiety aren't the same thing, that some people suffer badly with anxiety, and in those situations, it's not as simple as forcing yourself to do something. But personally, we have found that nine times out of ten, when you do something you've worried about a lot, you realise it wasn't so bad after all. Things are almost always worse in your mind than they are in reality, and knowing this can make you so much braver in life. Dancing has helped us learn that we could do whatever it was that we were scared of. We could overcome our fears. And if it doesn't go quite right? That's okay, too. Sometimes, you need to fail so you can learn.

We still get nervous. Whenever we're scared or worried about something, we push each other through these fears or rev each other up. It's helped a lot that we've had each other to go through those scary moments with.

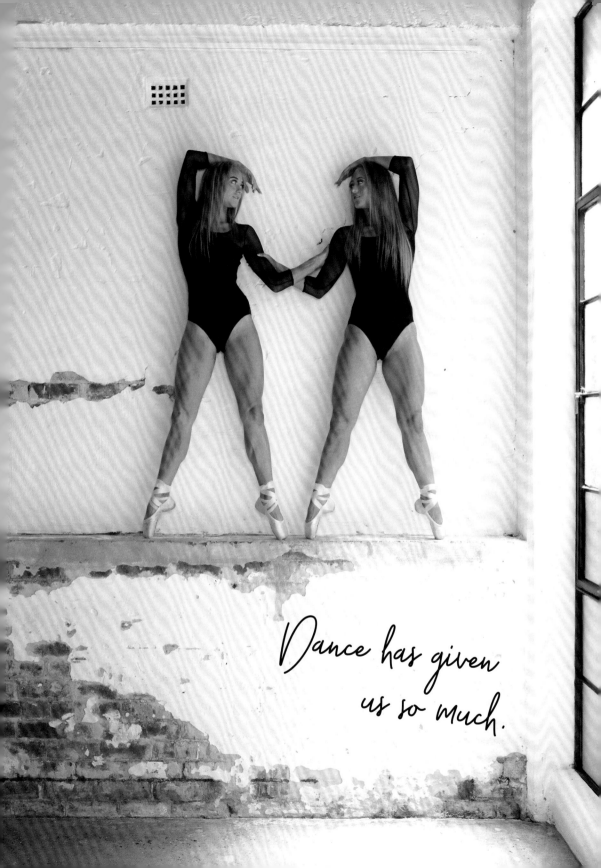

Dance has given
us so much.

# People actually know us?!

We were never the kids who said, 'I want to be famous.' It just never crossed our minds.

A note from ... *Sam*

> Well, actually, when I was young, I wanted to be a journalist (LOL! Even though public speaking was my worst nightmare). I guess in a way I'm doing a similar thing—I am talking to a camera every week!

We can't believe it when strangers on the street know who we are. We were in a flooring shop recently with Mum, and as soon as we walked in the guy working there pointed to us and said our names! Then he said, 'This may sound really weird, but I know exactly who you are. My wife watches you on YouTube.' People come up and ask us if we're the Rybka twins all the time. Not long ago, we were at the Sydney Harbour Bridge and a man came up to us to tell us that his daughters watch our videos. He could even tell the two of us apart! It was so unexpected—we loved hearing that his daughters watch us, and that he's watching along with them.

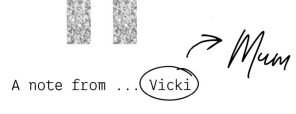

A note from ... (Vicki)  → *Mum*

Parents, it's good to be involved with your kids' online life. When kids are underage and on the internet, it's important to look out for them, keeping an eye on what they're doing and who they're interacting with.

The internet is a great tool, but it's also a place that can be negative and full of pressure. Parents should try to make sure that what their kids are doing is safe and not dangerous to them in any way. Watching videos with your kids, talking to them about who they follow and making sure you have access to their accounts is just a part of keeping them safe.

It's the coolest thing ever when dancers we admire and follow on social media know who we are. When we were travelling in the United States a few years ago, we were on Hollywood Boulevard doing the tourist thing. Suddenly, these girls started yelling out our names and running across the road to say hi to us. They turned out to be from the show *Dance Moms*—dancers from Candy Apple's. We love that show, so we totally knew who they were. They knew us through our social media, and we were like, 'You want to say hi to us? But you're the famous ones!' A year or two later, we ended up being part of a tour in Australia along with two of the girls from Candy Apple's, Haley Huelsman and Ashtin Roth, which was a fun coincidence.

Moments like this feel surreal to us, because in every other way, our lives are pretty much the same as always. We still own the same car that we had when we got our licences, we still live at home with our mum, we still go to dance classes, we still teach dance classes, we still love shopping and going to the beach with our friends, and we love our dogs, Buddy and Opie.

There's a lot more to us than dancing, Instagram and YouTube, and we're so excited that we get to share that stuff with you in this book. We're going to give you an insight into things that we don't necessarily share on social media, from how it really feels to be a twin, and how it feels to compete against each other, to why we love dancing as much as we do and how we decide which of us gets to wear something new first. Basically, we're going to answer those burning questions people have about our lives behind the scenes!

This book is our journey so far, but there's a lot more to come. We have so many more dreams to chase, and what we are going to do in the future changes from one day to the next. We never know who's going to come into our life, who the next email might be from, or what opportunity that might bring. It's a crazy roller-coaster ride— thank you for coming along on it with us. We hope you enjoy this part of our journey.

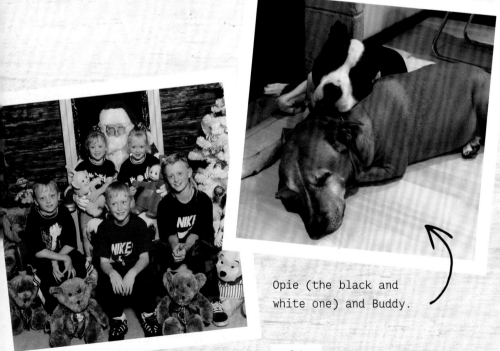

Opie (the black and white one) and Buddy.

Thank you for
coming on this crazy
ride with us!

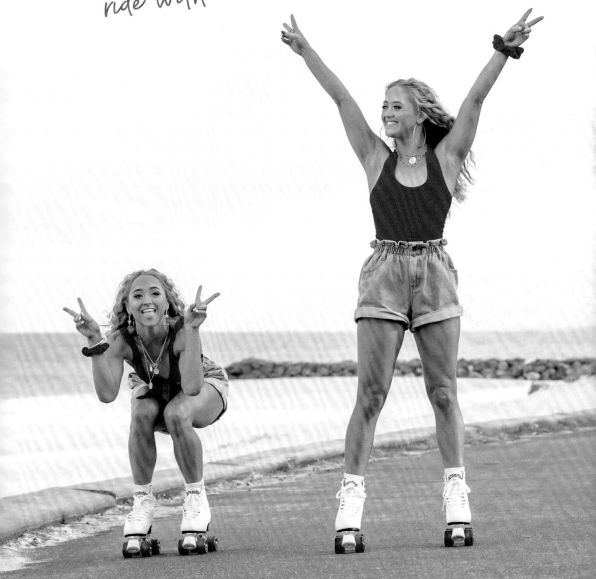

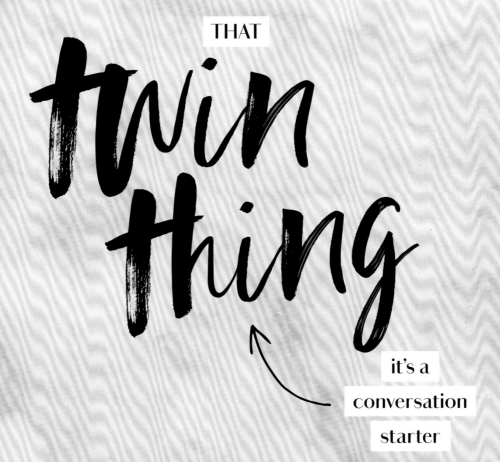

# CHAPTER 1

THAT

*twin thing*

it's a conversation starter

Being a twin is a natural conversation starter. When we were babies, people would stop our mum to ask about us, and now we often have strangers asking whether we are twins.

Through the years, many people have said things like, 'I wish I had a twin,' or 'I wonder what my twin would be like?' Being a twin just seems to be one of those things in life that a lot of people are curious about—although to us, it's the most natural thing in the world.

When it comes to people asking about our lives as twins, there are certain questions that come up again and again. Let's start with the easy ones.

## So, what's it like being a twin?

Our answer for this one is always the same: we don't know what it's like not to be a twin. The only way we can explain it is that it's like having your best friend with you all the time. (And how great is that?)

From our point of view, being a twin is the best thing in the world. Your twin always has your back. They know pretty much everything about you, and no matter what happens in life, good or bad, you've got them to go to. We can't imagine going through life without each other.

When it comes to things such as the first day of school, or going to a new dance class, we've always had each other.

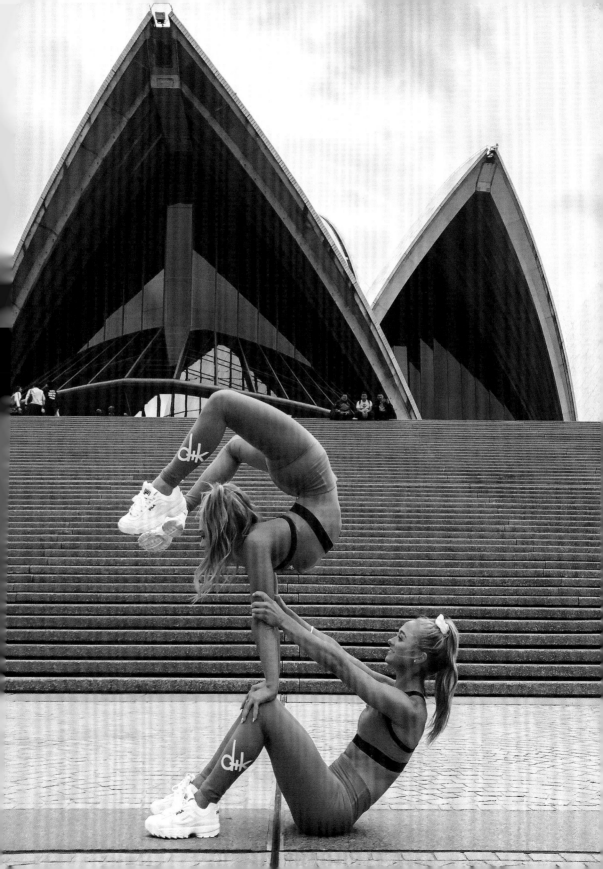

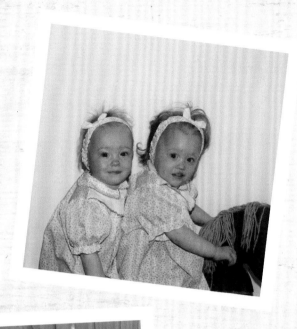

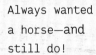
Always wanted
a horse—and
still do!

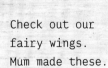
Check out our
fairy wings.
Mum made these.

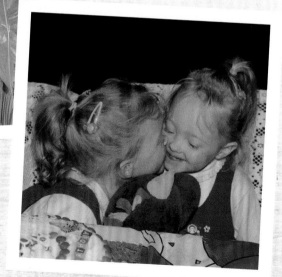

It wasn't until we got older that we realised how lucky we were. When you're younger, you don't analyse things too much—you just take them for what they are. But looking back, we realise how amazing it was that we had each other from day one. On those mornings when one of us was sick and had a day off school, it was scary for the other twin to have to go to school by herself. But it also helped us understand how other people feel when they are doing something new.

## Can you read each other's minds?

People always want to know whether twin telepathy is a real thing. So, can we actually read each other's minds? Well . . . yeah, in a way, but not because we are telepathic (at least we don't think we are!). But we are with each other every day, and always have been, so we find we have the same thoughts, and often the same thought process as well. Obviously, we have our own minds, but our thinking really is very close. Friends and family often tell us that we summarise things in a very similar way, too.

Once, when one of us was in a dance lesson, the other one told Mum about something that had happened earlier that day. When the other twin came out of their lesson and was alone with Mum, she told her the same story in the exact same way. Mum thought that was the craziest thing ever, but it just proves that our minds work in the same way. (It's funny how our mum has to listen to the same stories twice.)

Sometimes, our thoughts are so in sync that if there are a few moments of silence, we'll both say the same thing at the same time, or we'll suddenly start singing the exact same line of whatever song happens to be in our heads. And this isn't a one-off thing; it happens more than you might think.

# Do you wear matching outfits?

Yes and no. There's no denying that we have the same style and taste in clothes. The only thing that might be a little different is the colour scheme: Teagan is more of a girly girl, so she'll go for the pinks and rose golds, whereas Sam's into bright colours and is more out there. But when we go into shops, we usually like the exact same things, and we'll always pick the same styles or like the same clothes online. We have a rule that whoever sees something first, or picks it up first, gets to wear it first. But, because we like such similar things and we also like to coordinate with each other, there's always an option for the other person to wear something just as good as that new item anyway. Whenever we find one thing we like in a shop, we'll always try to find something similar to match it with.

*We decide on our outfits in the morning, and it's always a joint decision.*

...

If there's a big event coming up, we discuss our outfits to make sure they look good together. So Teagan might find a dress she loves, and then we'll try to find Sam a top and a skirt in the same colour or a similar pattern as the dress. That way, we're slightly different, but still coordinating. We don't like to wear the exact same thing, though; our outfits have to be different in style, colour or pattern.

When it comes to everyday clothes, we also like to coordinate with each other. We'll decide on our outfits in the morning, and it's always a joint decision. We'd love to say that it's smooth sailing, but it's not always the case—we are siblings, after all! And of course, sometimes we do wear matching outfits when we're having fun creating images for social media.

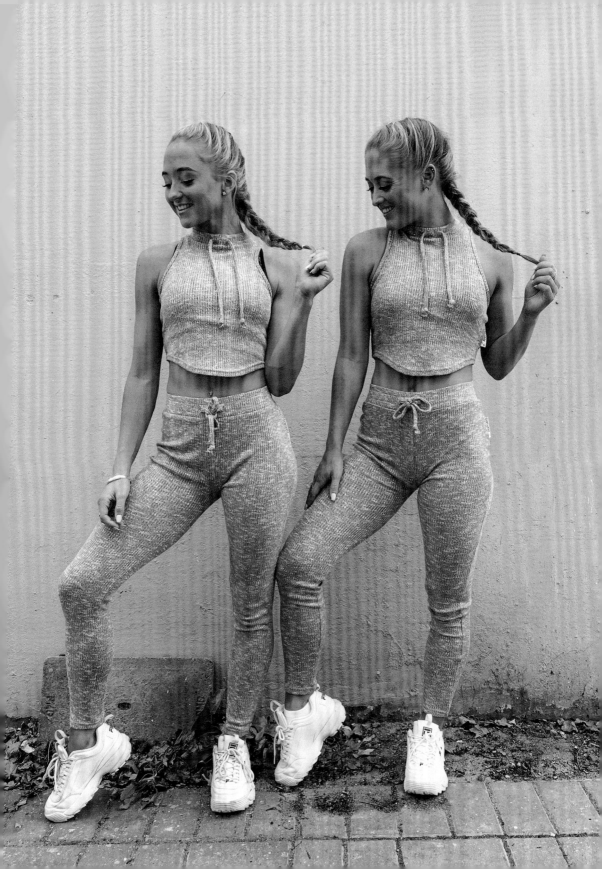

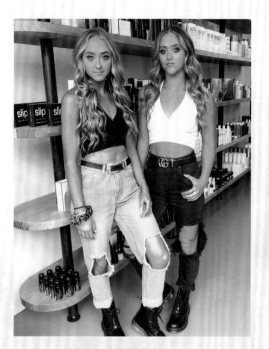
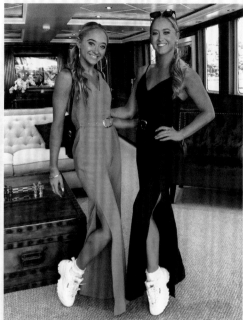

## Our approach to fashion

The thing we love most about fashion is how it helps us express ourselves. We can be whoever we want to be, showing our personalities through the clothes we wear. We really like summery vibes, so most of the time we keep things light and fun, with bright colours, pale pinks and frills. We try to stay on trend, experimenting with different looks and putting our own twists on them, and we like playing with edgier looks, depending on the event we're going to.

The world has changed so much. When we were younger, it felt as if everyone had different styles, but now that everyone's on social media, you can't help but be aware of the trends. And it feels like fashion has really stepped up—especially in Australia. When we travel to the United States, people often tell us they think Australians

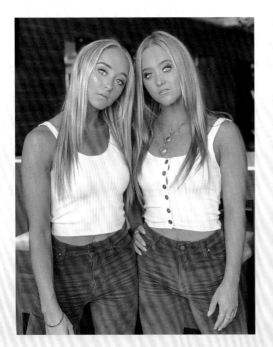
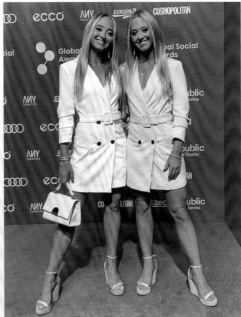

have great fashion sense. They also reckon our online stores are great, although they hate having to order from Australia because the clothes take so long to arrive.

People see our final looks on Instagram, but little do they know what went on before we settled on each outfit. We often try on about ten outfits before we're ready, and then usually end up going back to the very first one. (That's why our rooms get messy!) And even then, there are decisions about accessories: shoes, belts and bags.

We find the best way to get ready for an event with minimum fuss (and mess) is to envision what we want to wear before we start getting ready. Usually, if we do this and then put an outfit on, we're happy with it.

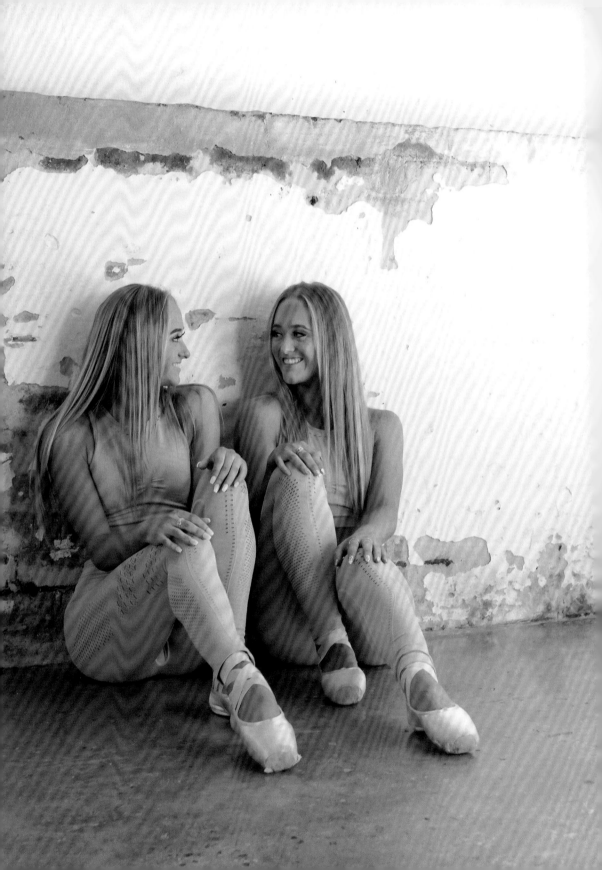

## Do you share everything?

Kind of! One thing that seems hard for people to believe is that we've only had our own bedrooms for a couple years now. We still live at home in the same house we grew up in. We shared a bedroom for 21 years, but when our older brothers moved out, we each got our own space. Sam stayed in our old room, and Teagan moved into the new room. This change was exciting for both of us, but so weird at the same time. Sleeping on our own after that many years in the one room took a lot of getting used to. We are both night people, so we stay up late (like, really late!). If one of us hears a noise at night, we'll grab our phone and text or call the other one right away: 'What was that noise? Was that you?!'

A note from ... *Teagan*

Still, to this day, I'll walk into our old room accidentally. Then I'll look around and think, oh wait, this isn't my room anymore!

Now that we're used to it, we love having our own rooms. And one of the nicest things about not sharing anymore is that we each get to design our own space.

*Your room is you!*

# Do you get separation anxiety?

Now we're getting into the deeper stuff. And the short answer is yes!

After we finished high school, we enrolled in the same degree at university: a Bachelor of Education in dance and drama, for teaching at high schools. This meant going to uni for four years. Naturally we took the exact same classes, lectures and tutorials. Not only did we get to experience uni together, but we were able to help each other out with big assignments, and that was a bonus. (It was like having two of yourself!)

But it wasn't all fun or straightforward. As part of our degree requirement, we had to complete a practical teaching element each year (aka, the 'prac'). During these pracs, we were placed at different high schools to get teaching experience. In the first year, the prac was three weeks long, but they got longer each year, ending with a massive ten-week placement in our final year.

*We learned so much and gained a lot of independence.*

•••

We were eighteen when we did our first prac placements, and this was the first time we'd ever been forced to separate from each other and focus on ourselves. Even driving alone to go to our different schools was strange! (We seriously do absolutely everything together, and we share a car.) Still to this day, those pracs were the only times in our lives we've spent completely on our own.

Being separated added a lot of extra stress and anxiety on top of the pracs, which were hard enough. Not having that other person to rely on or check things with was challenging. But we learned so much and gained a lot of independence during this time. We're glad we got to experience being apart, because it gave us an insight into what life must be like for people who aren't twins, and how it feels to brave new situations on your own. It's tough! But we got through it, and now we can each say, 'I did that, and I did it well.'

At the end of our pracs, we were both offered teaching jobs (together!) for the following year, which had been our original goal. But by that point, we'd promised to give ourselves a year off to focus on building our YouTube channel (more on that in Chapter 8), so we ended up turning down those jobs. If we do end up teaching in the future, though, we'd like to teach at the same school. For now, our passion is YouTube!

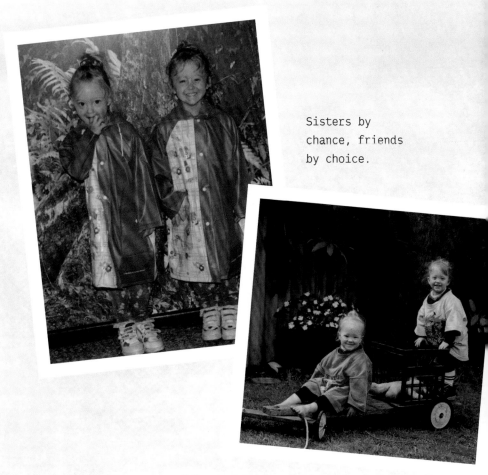

Sisters by chance, friends by choice.

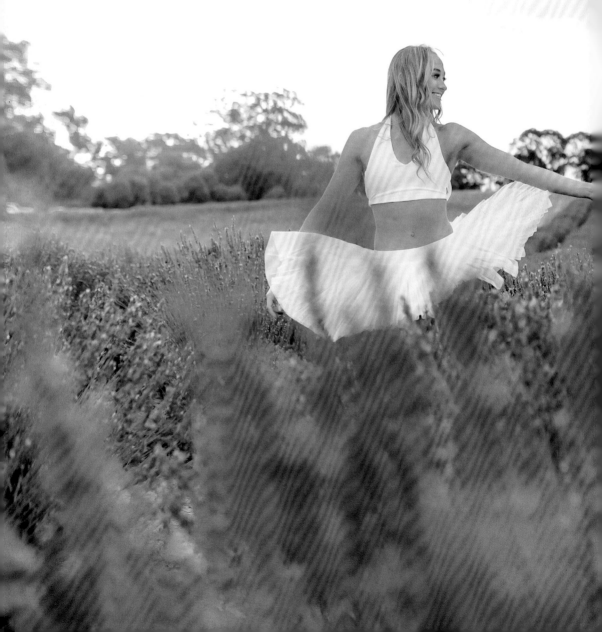

The greatest gift
our parents gave us

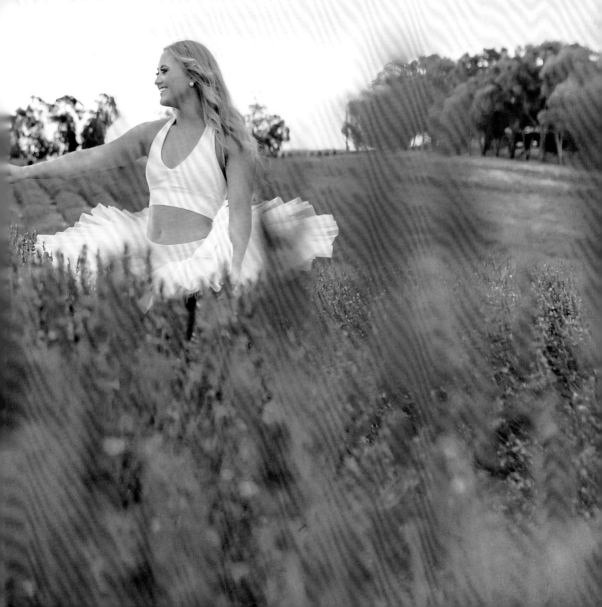

was each other.

# Do you ever want to be your own person?

Obviously, each of us is their own person, but we understand what people mean when they ask us this. Thankfully, we've never thought of being a twin as a bad thing. We've never wanted to separate our lives from each other, or felt the need to create distinct identities for ourselves, the way some twins do. In fact, the opposite is true: we are actually happy that we are so similar! We often think about how different things would be if one of us had loved dance and acro, and the other one hadn't. Lots of twins live completely different lives and have different likes, but we've always loved the same things.

The only negative thing about being so similar is that people are always comparing us with each other, trying to figure out which one is the smartest, the prettiest, the best dancer or the better acrobat. But that's probably true for most twins, most sisters and maybe even some best friends! Comparisons like this might push some siblings apart and make them competitive, but they've helped bring us closer and make us even better at what we do.

# Has competing against each other affected your relationship?

It's true that we've always been each other's natural competition, but rather than bringing each other down or trying to be better than the other, we've always focused on growing together and lifting each other up. We are our own healthy competition, always pushing ourselves to get better.

When we were younger, if one of us wasn't quite as good a dancer as the other, it would motivate us to work harder. That's probably why we are at the same level now, because we've pushed each other. When one of us gets a new trick, the other one thinks, 'I've got to get that now, too.' It's not in our nature to sit there and let the other one perfect a new move without striving to be as good as each other.

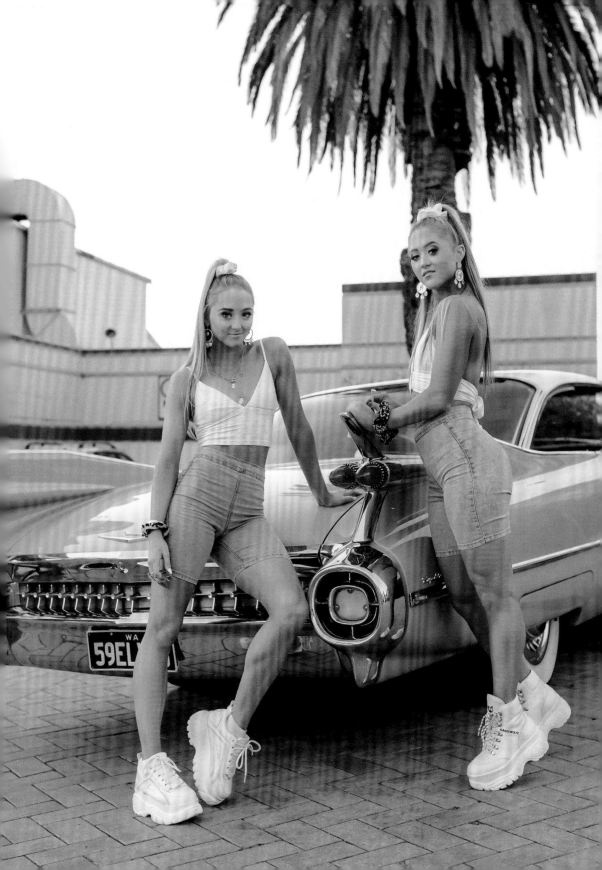

# Fairness is everything

We feel really lucky that we're able to be competitive with each other in this positive way. Without a doubt, this has everything to do with how we were raised.

All through primary school, Mum preferred us to be in the same classes. That way, she knew we'd have each other and could help each other out. Plus, when it came to making friends, it was probably easier for our parents if we had the same group of friends. But the main reason Mum wanted us in the same classes was that it was important to her that things were fair between us. Being in the same classes meant we couldn't say, 'Your teacher's better than mine,' or 'You've got nicer friends.' She kept us together so there wouldn't be arguments about those things. How could there be if we were having the same experiences?

*We have an agreement that when one of us wins, we share the prize.*

...

Mum and Dad always encouraged us to be fair with each other, and other people, and to give 150 per cent to whatever we do. They brought us up this way, and that's carried on in how we behave now.

Of course, when it comes to certain situations in life, such as competitions, there can only be one winner. And since we're the same age and the same skill level, we're always up against each other. But even in those situations, we find a way to keep things fair. For as long as we can remember, we've had an agreement that when one of us wins, we share the prize. Well, not if it's a trophy, but if it's money or a trip somewhere, we always share it. This feels right to us because we know that both of us have worked equally hard for whatever it is we are doing, so it's only fair that we both reap the rewards. Besides, a judge's decision is just that: one person's personal preference and opinion on the day.

When we compete, our goal is always to go out there and do the best that we can. Winning is just a bonus. We know that it's important to accept the judge's decision. Sometimes, no matter how hard you've practised or how much you want something, it just isn't your day. As long as we've tried our best, that's what matters.

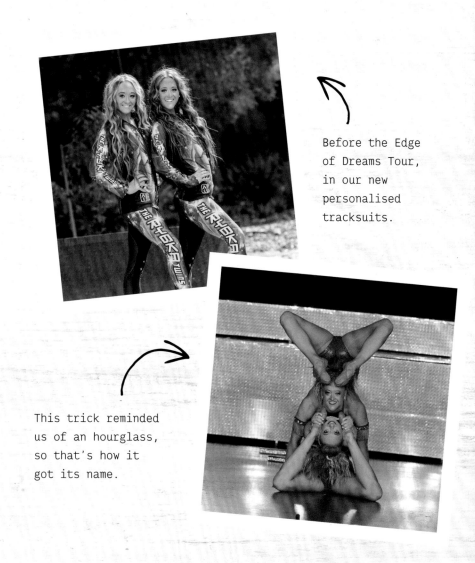

Before the Edge of Dreams Tour, in our new personalised tracksuits.

This trick reminded us of an hourglass, so that's how it got its name.

# CHAPTER 2

## Family first

O ur family is fairly big and getting bigger. There are five of us Rybka kids, and growing up as the youngest kids in a big family was a great experience. We had a really happy childhood. There's not a right or wrong way to raise kids, but we feel our parents did a great job. They were strict, but not too strict. And they always made sure that we had activities to focus on and goals to aspire to. We had our acro and dance classes from an early age, and each of our brothers had hobbies, too; they were always off doing sports such as football or camping or fishing with Dad.

## Mum's got our back

Both of our parents were very supportive, but when it came to dance and acro, Mum was in charge. It felt natural for her to do this, because she'd grown up dancing and doing acrobatics, too. She had a lot of experience and was at home in that world, so she was always more involved when it came to taking us to competitions and helping us practise our routines.

We wouldn't be where we are without our Mum. She's always been such a positive influence, standing behind us and motivating us to be as much as we can be, not just with dance, but with everything in life. Whenever we question something we are doing, she's there to reassure us, help us or remind us why we are doing it and what the bigger goal behind it is.

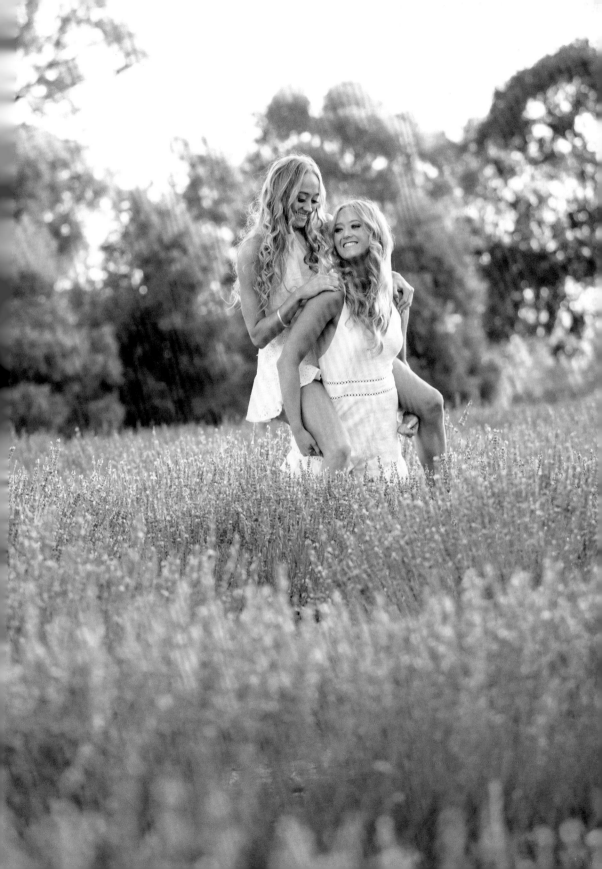

We are thankful that she's so good at acro, too! She's our personal acro coach and is always at the park when we practise. She watches us and tells us how things are going, so we get that critique when we're practising and not just in dance class. Over the years, all this extra coaching has helped us improve much faster.

Luckily for us, Mum loves being with us, and that we still live at home. We've got such a close relationship and feel grateful to have someone right there, in life and business, who wants the best for us.

When it comes to our YouTube channel and Instagram, Mum is our videographer and photographer. Without her, we'd struggle to produce the content we do. Whenever we travel, Mum is with us. She doesn't like being in our videos or photos, but she's always there, creating everything along with us. We've all learned so much on this journey, and we've learned it together. Like us, she always wants things to be as good as they possibly can be. She's our boss and our Mum. We often joke that she's like the third twin! If you watch our videos, you'll often hear Mum laughing in the background, and we love that we get a lot of comments from people saying they can hear her laughing.

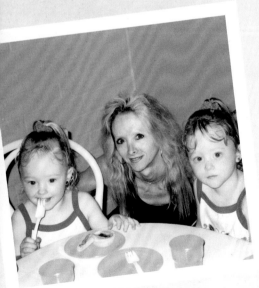

♡ Love you,
Mum!

Thanks for
everything
you do, Mum.

# Our dad: A true Aussie legend

Every Sunday when we were kids (about six or seven years old), we would all go as a family to watch our brothers' football games. This was an all-day event, and of course the two of us would take full advantage of the grass, cheering and doing acrobatics on the sidelines. The best part was asking Dad for money to buy lollies at the canteen. He'd always say, 'Only if you get me a meat pie.'

To people on the outside, it may have seemed like our father wasn't involved as much as our mum, but Dad was definitely there for us. Right from the beginning, he was our biggest supporter, always happy to fix or paint props for us—and he did a top job, too (thanks, Dad!). He made sure the front and backyard lawns were cut, watered and ready for us to practise our acro routines (even though his favourite line was 'Get off the lawn!').

## Right from the beginning, he was our *biggest supporter.*

• • •

Sadly, Dad is no longer with us. He passed away suddenly in 2017 and we didn't even get the chance to say a proper goodbye or tell him how much we loved him. But he was a legend in the eyes of so many people, including us. We couldn't believe how many people were at his funeral; it was a reflection of the type of man he was. It didn't matter who you were or what age you were or what job you did, Dad treated everyone as an equal. He was the friendliest person in the world, always ready with a smile and the world's strongest handshake.

Whenever Dad was around, we felt safe, as if nothing bad could happen. And if it did, he'd know what to do and how to sort it out. We always thought that if he got lost in the middle of the bush, he'd use his excellent skills to find his way out. He was a bit of a Crocodile Dundee in our eyes.

Dad was a true Aussie bloke from back in the day. He never owned a mobile phone (or even knew how to work one!). He didn't even use bank cards. And you could always hear Dad's vehicle coming from far away. It was one of a kind—just like him.

Mum used to tell us all the time how, whenever Dad met someone new, he'd ask whether they'd heard of 'the Rybka twins'. If they hadn't, he'd say, 'You can look 'em up on YouTube. They're my daughters.' We loved hearing this and loved knowing how proud of us he was.

Without fail, Dad came to each one of our end-of-year dance concerts, and before a competition, he'd be there to give us his famous words of encouragement, telling us to 'knock 'em dead', or 'show 'em how it's done' and to bring back a big trophy. When we came home at the end of a long competition day, we'd leave any trophies on the kitchen bench so they'd be the first things he'd see in the morning. We miss leaving those out for him, and we still hear his words of encouragement in our minds before every performance.

Our brothers' friends all loved Dad, too. When they got older, he'd sit and have drinks with them. He'd be the one giving them life advice or encouraging them about their jobs. He became a sort of father figure to many of them. After he passed away, some of our brothers' friends went up to where Dad used to fish to put a monument there for him. Others had little tribute items made—drink holders and hoodies, with words about what a legend Dad had been.

We are lucky to have so many happy memories of times with Dad, like going to the river with him when we were young and learning to fish, or staying up late at night and watching him fish with our brothers. He'll forever be the master of cooking the tastiest and biggest pancakes for Sunday breakfast, and the maker of the world's best deep-fried chips! A hug from him was like no other and we miss him every day.

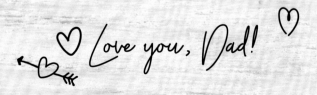

Love you, Dad!

# GRADUATION

When we graduated from university in 2016, our cohort included all the graduating classes across the Faculty of Education, not just our class. There were a lot of people in the convention centre that day: students, academic staff and the parents and family members.

One of the girls in our class had won the 'Dux', or top student, award. At the end of the graduation ceremony, she stood up to give her speech. We were sitting there, listening to her along with everyone else, when suddenly, we heard our names. We realised she was telling everyone our story! We looked at each other and said, 'She's talking about us!'

She talked about how we'd managed to stick with our dancing while going through university—how we'd managed to juggle things such as travelling, competing on *Australia's Got Talent* and making videos for YouTube while still giving 100 per cent to all our classes and assignments. Both of us were so shocked.

Our dad was there that day, and he couldn't believe that the top student was talking about us in front of all those people. It was an inspiring speech, and it felt amazing that Dad was there to hear it.

Christmas is easily one of our favourite times of the year!

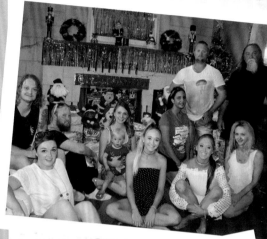

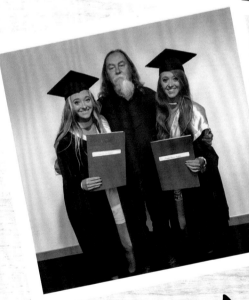

*We did it!*

# Yes, we have brothers!

A lot of people who know us, through social media or even as acquaintances, are shocked when they find out we have brothers—THREE of them!—Mitchell, Cody and Clayton. (We sometimes get asked about our parents' first names, too. The answer is Vicki and Steve.) Even though our brothers aren't on social media much, they definitely exist. They tend to be a bit camera-shy when it comes to being 'out there' on social media. Because of this, even dance friends who see us regularly with our mum often assume it's just the three of us.

Growing up with three older brothers was the best. They've always been extremely protective of us, and we liked that. Mitchell, the oldest, was the most protective. As kids, if we were ever crying or upset about anything, he'd be the first one there trying to sort it out.

As protective as he was, Mitchell enjoyed throwing us in the pool a lot! Because he was the oldest, and therefore the strongest, he also liked carrying us around by our ankles. He'd hold us upside down and get us to test our strength by trying to touch our toes. It was silly and fun, and probably great training now that we think back on it.

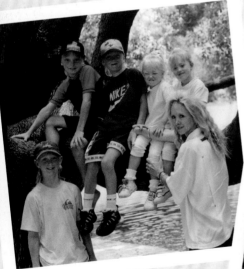

Growing up with older brothers was the best.

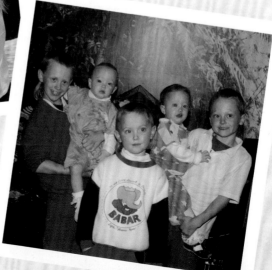

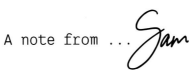

## A note from ... *Sam*

I developed this weird fear for a short time when I was seven where I was suddenly scared to do a bend-back. I don't know how or why it happened, but out of nowhere, after years of doing that trick with no issues at all, I just couldn't do it.

I was standing in the kitchen with Mum and Teagan, and we were all talking about it—I was probably getting a bit upset—and Mitchell heard us. He came in and said, 'Sam, what's the matter?' When I told him, he said, 'A bend-back? Even I can do that!' He whipped out this bend-back right there in the kitchen, from standing! We had no idea he could do that—Mitchell probably wasn't 100 per cent sure he could do it either, but he wanted to help. If he could prove to me that he could do a bend-back, then maybe I'd realise it was no big deal, and I'd be able to do it again, too. It was pretty funny, and you know what, it actually did help!

Even though our brothers were into fishing and sports, they'd often join in with us and do acro and stuff like that when we were at home. There was always some sort of competition going on in our games room. We'd be in there practising tricks or having headstand competitions during the TV ad breaks. The youngest of our three brothers, Clayton, was really good at headstands—he could hold them for a long time. Our goal was to try to beat him by holding ours for longer. Cody, our middle brother, would also do them. But it was always just fun for them; something to do while we hung out at home.

As it turns out, Mitchell wasn't the only brother with undercover acro skills. Not that long ago, we were all standing around in the kitchen talking about walking on our hands when Clayton casually said, 'Oh, I can do that.' And right there, in our kitchen (which isn't the biggest, by the way), he just popped up into a handstand. We were shocked out of our minds! He didn't even hit any furniture. Afterwards, he was like, 'Yeah, I used to do those at school all the time.' All those years growing up, our brothers must have been perfecting our acro moves while we weren't looking. Who knew they were that good?

## There's always time for family

As we got older, our brothers started moving out of the house one by one. This was a big adjustment. It's much quieter without them around, and there's more food in the fridge, but we don't get to laugh and hang out with them as much as we used to. The upside is that we get to be aunts to their amazing kids (plus Teagan inherited one of their bedrooms—cheers, Cody!).

But even with all of them gone, and all of us busy with our own lives, we've managed to stay close. We're lucky because our brothers live near enough that we still get to see them and their families often. Cody has done lots of travelling, and for a while he even wanted to live in Canada. But now that our other brothers have kids, he's come back and we can all be near each other again. Mitchell is now a commercial plumber, Cody is an electrician and Clayton is a domestic plumber.

Rather than try to schedule time to catch up whenever people are free, we have a regular family get-together every other Tuesday. Some people might think that doesn't sound often enough, but those Tuesday nights come around quickly. When we do get together, it's a madhouse; there are kids everywhere.

We feel that family is so important. No matter what craziness is going on in your life, you can always come back to family. To them, we are always just Teagan and Sam.

## Aunts in training

We have five nieces and nephews. The oldest is three, and the youngest (twins) are eight months old. Yep, that's right: more Rybka twins! Clayton and his wife, Ash, already had two little ones—a girl and a boy—when they found out they were having twins: a girl and a boy! It was the biggest, craziest surprise, but also so cool.

We love being aunts and watching all the kids grow up and become their own little people. It's kind of funny: because we were the babies in our family, we weren't used to being around young children. When it came to handling or holding a baby, we weren't that confident. If we're being completely honest, we used to be kind of scared of babies! But now, we've had lots of practice, and we love being around our brothers' kids because they're so into everything. As our nieces and nephews are all still so young, we normally babysit with our mum (aka Nana Vic). Since she's the one with all the baby experience, she deals with most of the hard stuff, like changing nappies or settling, but we love to help. Having these new relationships has taught us that you don't have to know what you're doing—you just kind of figure things out as you go along.

Clayton's little girl, Ella, who's almost two, sees us dancing all the time, so we're hoping she'll want to try dancing when she's older. And we're guessing that Harlem, Mitchell's son, is going to be a hip-hopper. He has a natural swag about him—he's a little rebel! Even if our brothers don't put them into dancing, we'll probably try to sneak a few private lessons in at home so they can give it a go. They might absolutely love it. You never know!

We love spending time with our nieces and nephews.

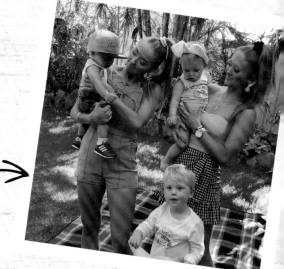

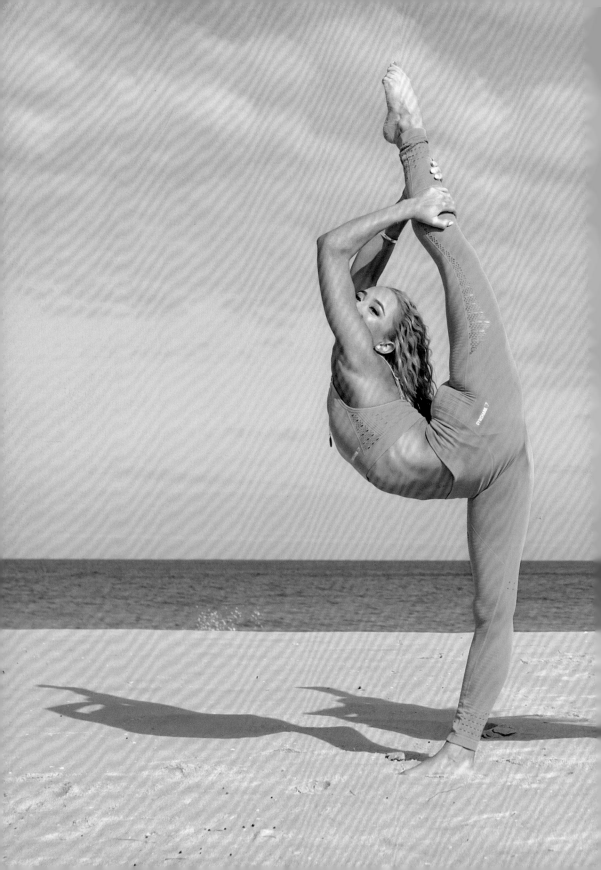

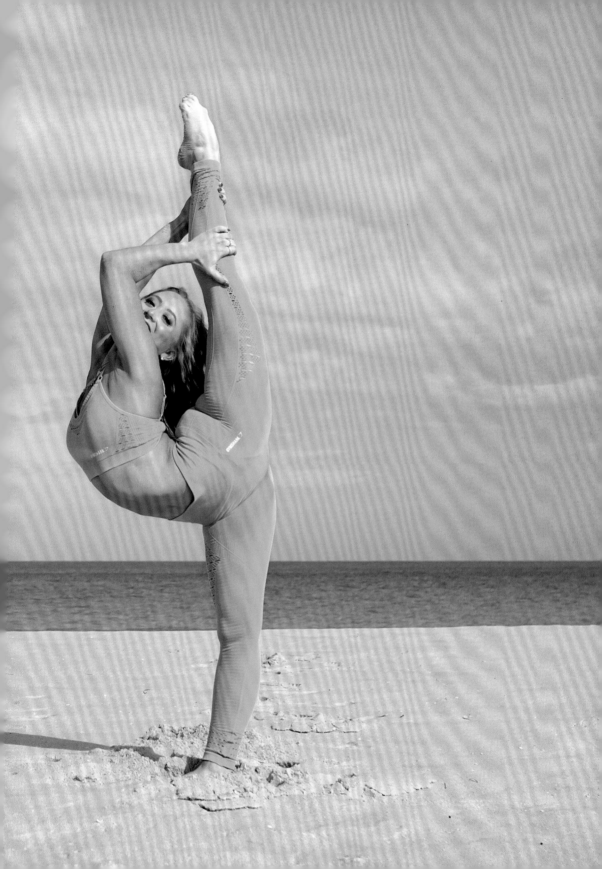

# CHAPTER 3

# Friends
## MAKE OUR
# world go
# 'round

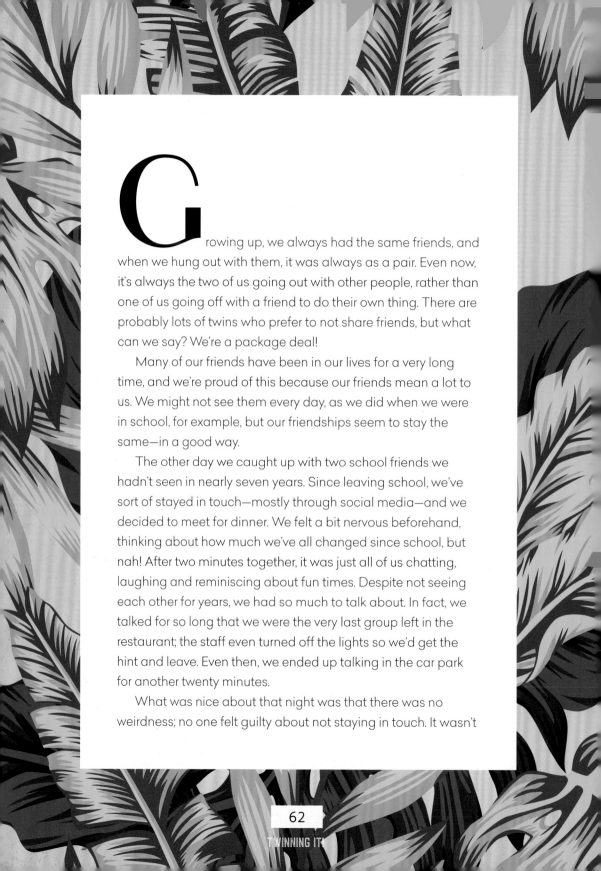

Growing up, we always had the same friends, and when we hung out with them, it was always as a pair. Even now, it's always the two of us going out with other people, rather than one of us going off with a friend to do their own thing. There are probably lots of twins who prefer to not share friends, but what can we say? We're a package deal!

Many of our friends have been in our lives for a very long time, and we're proud of this because our friends mean a lot to us. We might not see them every day, as we did when we were in school, for example, but our friendships seem to stay the same—in a good way.

The other day we caught up with two school friends we hadn't seen in nearly seven years. Since leaving school, we've sort of stayed in touch—mostly through social media—and we decided to meet for dinner. We felt a bit nervous beforehand, thinking about how much we've all changed since school, but nah! After two minutes together, it was just all of us chatting, laughing and reminiscing about fun times. Despite not seeing each other for years, we had so much to talk about. In fact, we talked for so long that we were the very last group left in the restaurant; the staff even turned off the lights so we'd get the hint and leave. Even then, we ended up talking in the car park for another twenty minutes.

What was nice about that night was that there was no weirdness; no one felt guilty about not staying in touch. It wasn't

We didn't realise
we were making
memories, we just
knew we were
having fun.

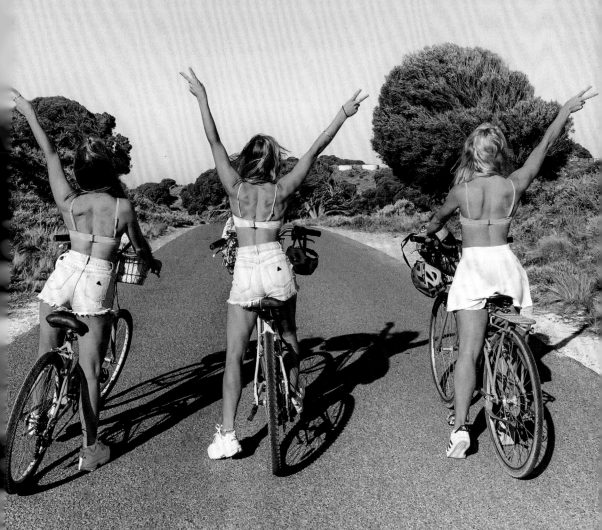

anything bad, it was just that we all got busy going to uni, getting jobs, earning money … living the adult life. It happens!

That dinner reminded us that it's always worth reconnecting with people who've meant a lot to you in the past. No matter how much your life might change, you shouldn't ever forget those people who've been there for you. These girls were our good friends all through school, which was an important time in our lives. They knew us before we were on TV and YouTube, before we had followers and fans. We know that they like us for us, and that counts for a lot.

Friendship isn't just about who you've known for the longest. It's about who walked into your life, and said "I'm here for you".

## Friends in two worlds

During our school years, our lives were split between two different worlds: school and dance. Because of that, we've always had two distinct groups of friends: our school friends and our dance friends.

Our school friends were, and still are, so important to us. When you're in school, everything that happens feels so important and dramatic, and your friends ride that roller-coaster with you. They're a big part of who you are during those years. But, as close as we were to our school friends, we had a very different—and in some ways deeper—connection with our dance friends.

Our dance friends felt more like family. We had so much in common with them, and we could be more ourselves around them. It's hard to say why. Perhaps it's because we spent so much more time with them, or maybe we just got lucky. Many of our dance friends were a bit younger than us. But that didn't make any difference to us. In our eyes we were all equal. At school, age seems so important, but after school, it feels like everyone is the same age. It just doesn't matter that much any more.

For most of our lives, we kept these two groups of friends pretty separate. When we did bring them together, they didn't seem to mix that well—not that they didn't get along, just that it was a little harder

# don't let school drama destroy you

What goes on at school can feel like such a big deal at the time, and it is a big deal when you're going through it. But no matter what, don't let what happens at school destroy you as a person. Once you're done with school, no one is going to ask what group you were in. Of course, when you're at school that stuff might seem important, but trust us, after school, nobody cares!

Let us 'Cher' a little wisdom with you. We love this quote from the singer Cher (and we love her, too). It's something her mum told her:

## 'If it doesn't matter in five years, it doesn't matter.'

65

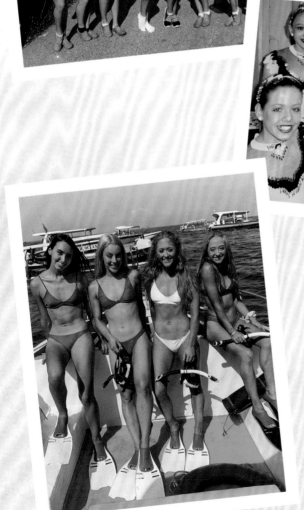

We value time with
our friends. Good
times and crazy
friends make the
best memories.

because we were all young, and they had different interests. Now that we're older, we've been bringing our different friends together more and more, and they get on well. And why wouldn't they? They're all warm, friendly people who are welcoming to others.

Now we feel more comfortable inviting our old friends out with new people, and bringing our uni friends and dance friends together (although, to be honest, our two best uni friends also happen to be dancers, so they're technically dance friends, too!). Seeing these different groups connecting with each other is so nice. Guess it's a perk of getting older!

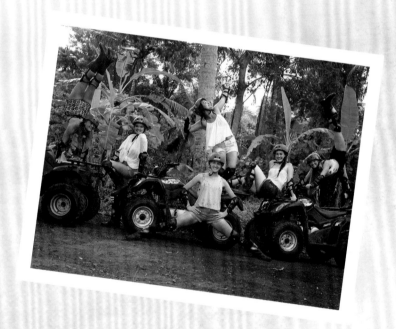

# Find good friends, then keep 'em

All this talk about different groups might make us sound like social butterflies, but we believe that when it comes to friends, it's quality over quantity. We've never cared about having as many friends as possible, or needing to be part of a certain group. We just want to be surrounded by people who lift us up, and who we can lift up, too. If someone doesn't make us feel good, we don't stick around just to add another friend to the list.

When it comes to meeting new people, the two of us are usually on the exact same page. Thankfully, there's almost never been a person that one of us liked and the other one didn't. Here are the top traits we look for in a friend. How does your bestie measure up?

A good friend should be ...

- supportive and encouraging
- down-to-earth
- someone who never drags you down or makes you feel bad about yourself
- accepting of who you are during good and bad times
- a good listener
- someone you have FUN with
- someone you can be yourself with.

And, of course, everything that we look for in a friend, we hope to be for our friends, too.

# When you make a new friend ...

How good is it when you meet someone
new but feel as if you've been friends
for years, or maybe you knew each other
in another lifetime (spooky!)? And if
you share a similar sense of humour,
that's the best. Being able to laugh
at anything and everything together
means that every time you catch up,
you just know you're going to make
awesome memories.

*Friends are the family we choose for ourselves.*

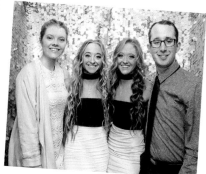
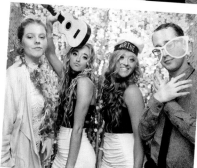
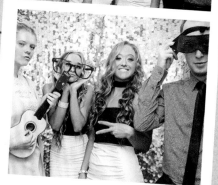

# Make time to be a good friend

If you want to have strong friendships that last, you've got to make time, no matter how busy you are. Everyone's life gets busier as they get older, but you can always find time for a quick catch-up or to connect in some way—whether that's liking their Instagram posts or sending them a funny text. You don't ever want your career to take over your friendships or other important relationships in your life.

As your world grows beyond school and uni, it's important to keep making new friends who understand those other aspects of your life, too. This has happened for us—we've even started making friends through social media. There have been people we've followed on Instagram or YouTube for a while, and when we met them, we already knew so much about their lives that the relationship didn't feel new or strange at all. We just connected straight away.

When good things happen in your life, true friends will always be happy for you. Most of our close friends are hugely encouraging and supportive, and we're thankful for that. They show so much interest, always remembering stuff we've told them and asking, 'How's that going?' or 'What's next?'

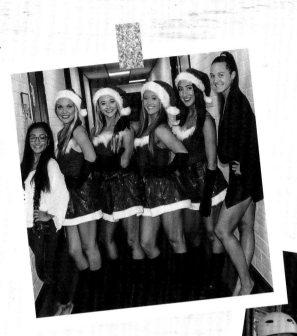

Time with friends creates
memories that stick with
you forever—big things and
small things, crazy things
and fun things!

Always up for an
adventure with
these girlies ...
especially in Bali!

# Unexpected friends

When you're in the dance world, especially on the competition circuit, you tend to see the same people every few months, and you can end up competing against the same dancers for many years. Instead of staring each other down from across the stage, we'd often go over to other dancers to say hi and have a chat. And because of that, we became quite good friends with a lot of the girls and boys in our group. We'd look forward to seeing them at the next comp because, even though they were our competition, we had built good relationships with them. We still see many of them now at competitions, workshops and classes.

When it comes to competing, of course you should be competitive when you're onstage. But when you're offstage, you should be friends. You don't have to carry that competitive energy into how you deal with each other offstage. We'd much rather be friends and make connections with other dancers. After all, we are there for the same reasons, and because we love the same thing. We have so much in common with other dancers, so we prefer to make the competition experience a positive one, rather than add extra stress. This is probably one of the major reasons we looked forward to competing so much. For us, it was never a negative thing.

One of our biggest rules in life is to be kind to everyone. When you first meet someone, you never know what might come from that one encounter or relationship. You also never know what that person might be going through in their life at that moment. We're big believers of the idea that everyone is equal; no amount of trophies or followers on social media will make you better than anyone else.

## Relationship talk

Most people crush on someone at some point, so naturally, we're often asked if either of us is in a relationship, and what type of qualities we look for in a partner. It's pretty simple! We look for someone who is …

*Honest*

*Kind*

*Funny*

*Motivated*

*Understanding*

*Genuine*

*Supportive*

That said, finding that special someone isn't an easy thing to do! We've never gone on any dating apps or websites because we feel the best way to meet people is in person—you never know who that person behind the screen might be. We'd always rather get to know someone in person and know that a person likes us for us.

When we were younger, we spent so many years consumed with dance that we never thought much about dating that. Now that we're older, we're both ready for relationships. We often talk about how awesome it would be if we could find twin boys to date. How funny would that be! But even though we know so many twin girls, we know hardly any twin boys.

73

Whatever happens, even when we have our separate lives, we know that we'll live close to each other (a street away would be perfect). And we'll always work together, so we'll get to see each other every day that way, too.

**When it comes to dating, there are certain rules that we live by:**

- **Look out for red flags!** If something seems wrong or 'off', don't just dismiss it.
- **Listen to close friends and family.** They might tell you things you don't want to hear, but always remember that they're the ones who know you the best. They've got your best interests at heart. If they don't like the person you're in a relationship with, that's a big red flag!
- **Never let someone change who you are.** If you can't be yourself, that's not a healthy relationship.
- **Never ditch your friends.** It doesn't matter how great your relationship might be, you still need girl power (or guy power—guys can be great friends, too!) in your life. Your friends are always there for you, so don't ever burn those bridges. The same goes for your family. Never push them aside for a relationship; they are all-important.
- **Go into new relationships slowly.** No matter how good something seems at the beginning, it takes time to know if you can trust a person.

It's important to follow your heart, but not if it compromises too many things you believe in. You should never lower your standards when it comes to the type of person you want in your life. Obviously, nobody is 'perfect', so you can't be too hard on someone you are in a relationship with, but, at the same time, it's important to stay true to your values. You should be treated well by the people close to you—don't lower those expectations for the sake of a guy. All the things you expect from a good friend, you should expect from the person you're in a relationship with, too.

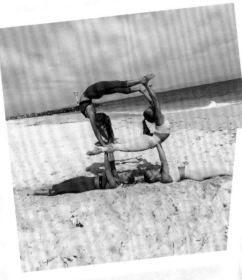

Friends that dance together, stay together.

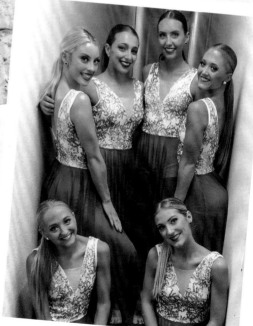

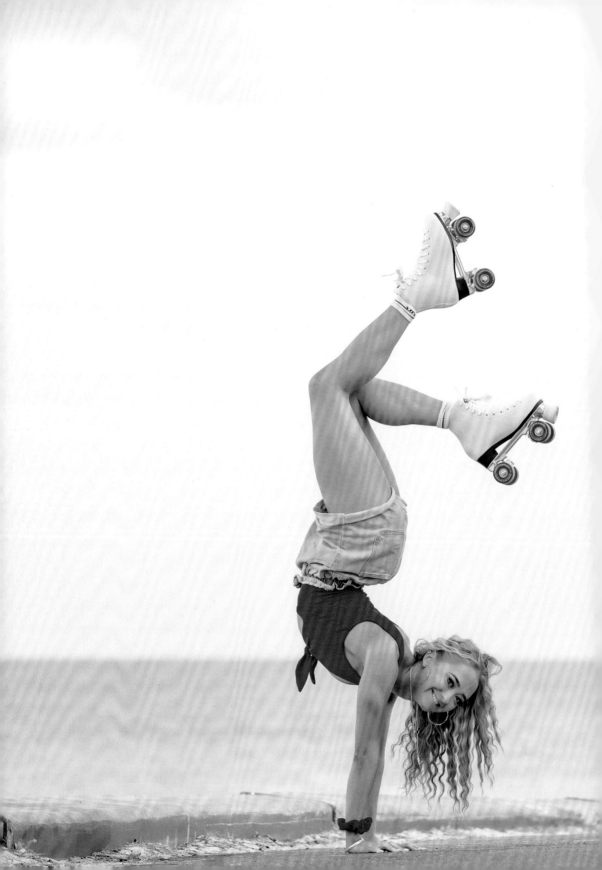

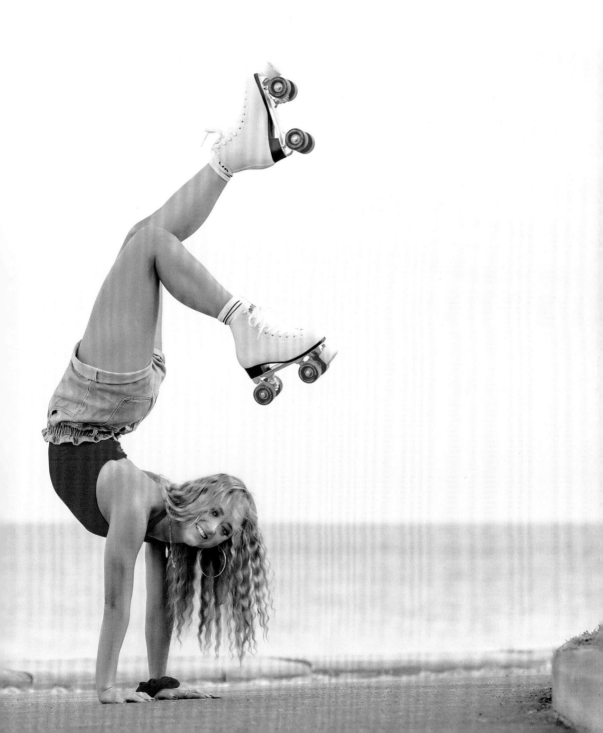

# CHAPTER 4

# Acro, dance AND competitions

T here's a saying we see a lot and it goes something like this: 'Find something you love, and you'll never work a day in your life.' We're not sure who said it first but whoever it was, they're right. We love this quote. It feels so true for us, especially now. It also reminds us how grateful we are that we found the thing we love doing when we were little. It's hard to imagine our lives without dancing. It's been a part of us for as long as we can remember.

Mum put us in our first acro class when we were three years old, and from the moment we did our first forward rolls, we loved it. That class wasn't serious at all, and there was no pressure or master plan to turn us into competitive dancers. Mum just wanted us to love acro and dancing, like she had growing up. She took a casual approach and found a school that she felt suited us best. It was a more relaxed environment than some of the other schools and wasn't all go, go, go!

Mum is our very own 'dance mom'! She had a long history with dance and acro before we came along, so she knows so much about that world. As a little girl with older sisters who danced, she grew up around dance classes—hanging out in the studio before she was out of nappies, and starting her first proper classes at three. She and her friend Debra McCulloch (who ended up being our teacher later on) grew up dancing together. They also performed as duo partners. Back then, they didn't have dance competitions the way we do, but they did

Sometimes life
appears to be upside
down, but as long as
you have someone
upside down with
you, you'll be okay.

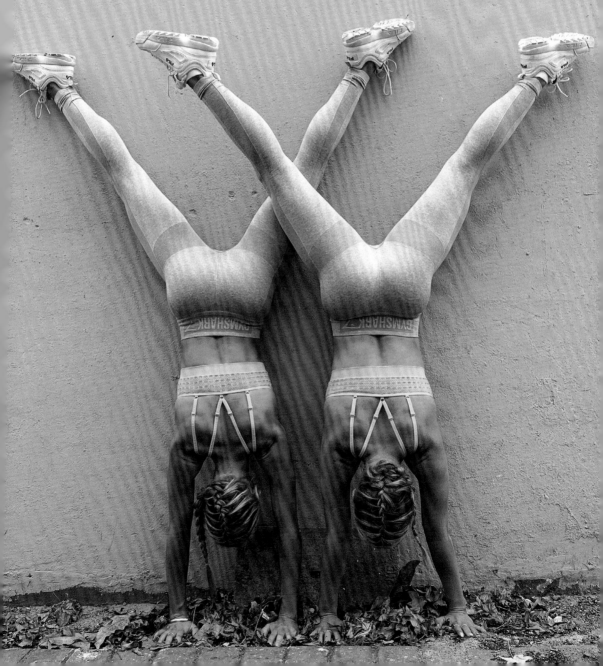

have floor shows. When Mum was six or seven, she'd do the shows with the older girls. They'd just put her out on stage for the quick work, like tumbling, because she was good at it. When most kids her age were home in bed, Mum was out performing.

Because Mum had loved growing up around acro and dance so much, she wanted to introduce us to that world so we could experience it, too. As much as Mum wanted us to like dance, it was really important to her that we make our own decisions about whether or not to continue with lessons. When we were almost six, Mum put us into a basic jazz dance class. Again, it was all about us having fun. Just like acro, we loved dancing right away, and because we were so into acro by this point, we also continued taking those classes. In fact, we did acro at home, on the beach, in the park ... We'd have done it every single day for hours on end if we'd been able to. Being capable of doing tricks, such as a cartwheel or bend-back, was so cool.

From that point, we added on an extra dance class each year along with acro—experimenting with different dance styles one by one. Jazz one year, tap the next, then ballet after that ... there were so many styles to explore. Mum made sure we took things slowly. We didn't even take ballet until we were nine, which is probably later than the average dancer. But she didn't want us to burn out.

Throughout our lives, it never crossed our minds to give up our dance classes. We never questioned for a minute whether to go to dance, or why we had to do it. We just did it and loved it. Each year, when enrolment time came around, we were the ones asking Mum, 'Okay, what can we try next? Can we do ballet this year? How about tap?' We wanted to do more and more. There was no question that we had found our niche.

After a couple years, our first dance school closed, so Mum had to move us to another dance school. She put us into Debra McCulloch Dance Academy, and we absolutely loved our new school. We practically grew up there between the ages of seven and twenty.

The dance studio will always be like a second home to us. The memories we made there are so special. Our dance friends were

'Find something
you love,
and you'll never work
a day in your life.'

— Unknown

Truth Bomb

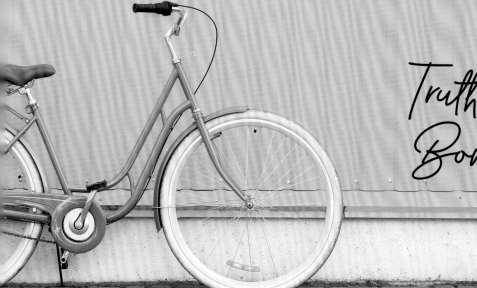

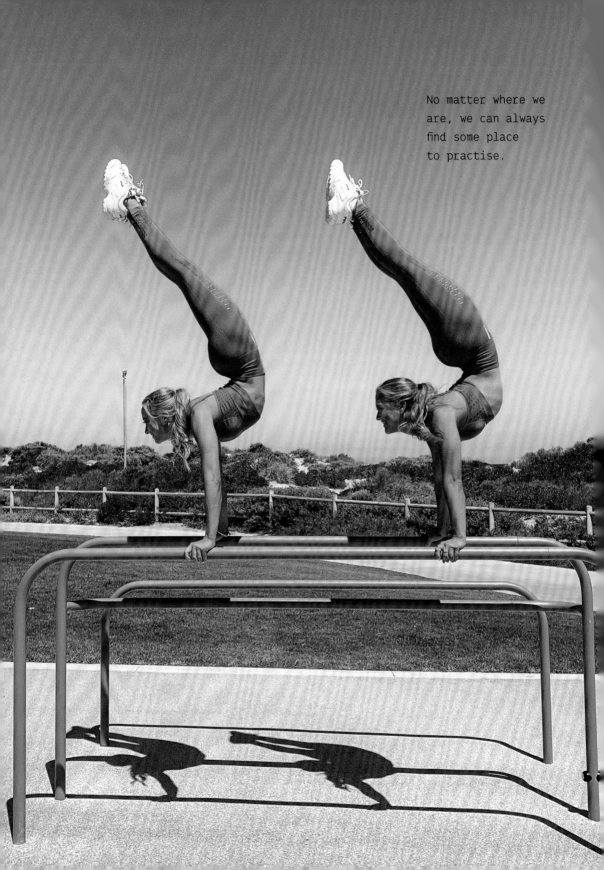

No matter where we
are, we can always
find some place
to practise.

down-to-earth and completely on the same wavelength as us. Each of us wanted to be there, we all loved dancing and we all had that passion in common. The two of us never had a day off from dance unless we were really, really sick.

## Acro

If you've been wondering what this 'acro' thing we keep talking about is, we're going to explain right now! Acro is like gymnastics. The difference is in how you train, how you execute the moves and the work, and the overall look of the performance. Gymnasts work on a spring-loaded floor for optimal rebound and protection during challenging tumbling passes. Acro is designed to go hand-in-hand with dance training, so it is usually taught in a dance studio with a sprung floor. This helps with shock absorption.

While gymnasts use apparatus, such as beams and bars, in acro there's no use of apparatus, although sometimes you do use props or do partner work—for example, when several students join together to create human pyramids or to make creative patterns.

Gymnasts will perform a powerful run into a trick, but an acro dancer performs a more lyrical dance step to transition into a trick. Most people describe gymnastics as a sport and acrobatics as an art. As dancers, we feel that acro is great for developing extra strength to enhance your ability to leap and turn in your technique classes.

There are three main components in acro: contortion, balancing and tumbling. Everyone is naturally better

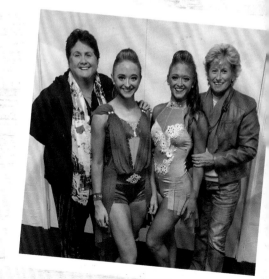

Miss Deb (left) and Miss Roche—not just our teachers, but our family!

at one aspect than the others. We've always had strong arms (at least according to Mum), so the balancing component came fairly naturally to us. Even so, we struggled with certain balancing moves and had to work at those. But the area we had to work the hardest for was contortion. Some kids can drop down into splits the first time they try them—they're built that way. Those kids will probably find the contortion element of acro easy, whereas less flexible dancers will have to work extra hard to catch up to them.

Mum was one of those super-flexible kids. There are pics of her doing contortion tricks when she's really young, and her butt is on her head! Anyone looking at those photos would probably assume that we had the same natural abilities as her, but that wasn't the case.

We were completely average in that department and have had to work very hard to achieve the levels of flexibility we needed to be classified as contortionists. We're always saying, 'Mum, why didn't you give us that flexibility gene?' (We must have our Dad's back!)

With our splits, we weren't flat straight away. We had to work at it, especially on our middle split and our non-preferred leg. Sometimes these things take a while. When you're working on your flexibility, take it slow. You can't rush things—that's how you get hurt.

Mum makes it
look so easy.

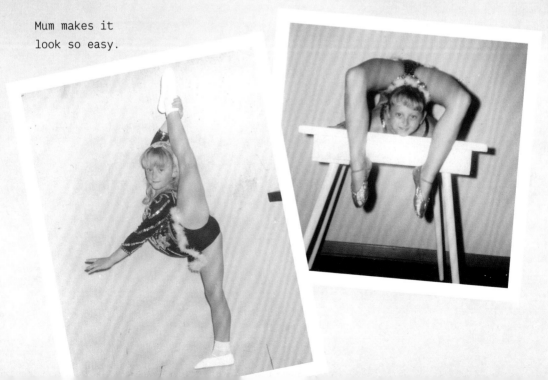

It's a long process when you do it safely; it's okay to push yourself, but you shouldn't expect results quickly.

We remember going to our room and sitting in the splits on our beds for as long as we could to improve our flexibility. Even though we'd been taking acro classes since we were three, it wasn't until we were about fourteen that we could be classified as proper contortionists. Before then, we could do general acro tricks but not all contortion tricks. We consistently worked on building our flexibility and kept pushing ourselves gently. Gradually, we were able to push our backs just that little bit more. Eventually, we were able to do other tricks that we'd never been able to do before.

You can always *improve* as long as you are *determined* and willing to *work hard*.

• • •

Today, people see us doing certain moves and ask, 'Does that hurt?' The truth is, there are little pinches here and there. After all, we are pushing our backs and bodies to do things most bodies don't do. But if you warm up correctly and are careful, it shouldn't hurt—especially if you've trained for the tricks. If you're working on building up a particular physical aspect and have trouble pushing past a certain threshold, just remember that it doesn't matter how old you are; even if you've been doing something since you were young, you can always improve as long as you are determined and willing to work hard.

In a way, we even think it's better that we had to work hard to get our bodies to this point. If things had come too easily, perhaps we wouldn't have the work ethic we do now. We proved to ourselves that if we work and work, we can achieve our goals.

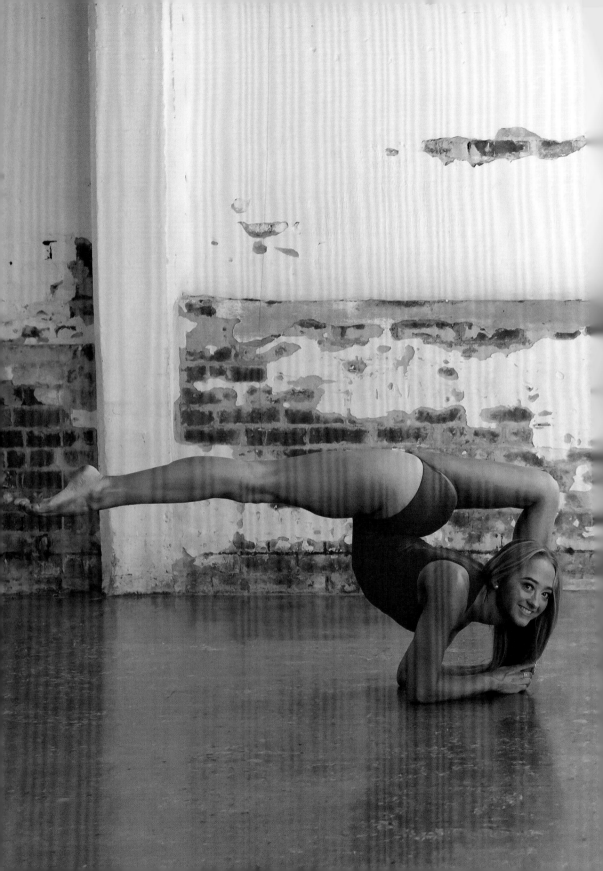

*We had to work very hard
to achieve the levels of
flexibility we needed.*

# The styles of dance

If you love dancing so much that you want it to be a career, it's better to have experience in all genres. It's not uncommon to go to an audition and have them say, 'Okay, great ballet technique, but now I need to see an aerial.' If you can do an acro trick as well as ballet, or whatever else they happen to ask for, you've got more of a chance at making it through to the next round.

We've found that every dance style helps or crosses over in some way to another genre:

## Dance styles

**Hip-Hop** Great for getting grounded as a dancer, and it therefore helps with commercial jazz, because you have to be more grounded when dancing in that style. It also helps with isolating parts of the body, which is so important in commercial jazz, lyrical and contemporary. The ability to isolate and move parts of your body—your chest, shoulders or whatever else—in weird, crazy ways helps in all genres.

**Jazz** Jazz is more technical than hip-hop. It uses lots of fancy kicks, leaps and spins, which can go in pretty much any genre of dancing.

**Tap** There are so many different styles of tap now. We learned theatrical tap (old-school tap!), which helped us with arm lines and head lines, musicality and rhythm.

But perhaps none of these styles helps or improves you more as a dancer or acrobat than **ballet** …

90

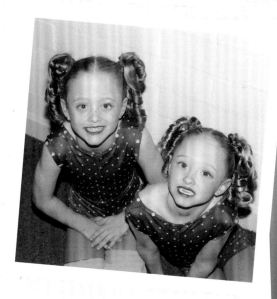

Dancing is the
closest thing to magic.

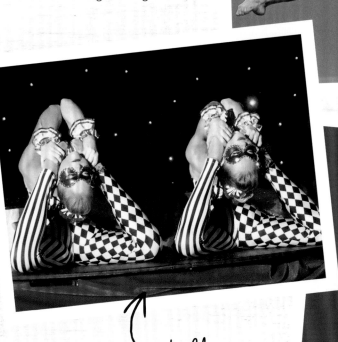

Fringe World
Festival in Perth

ACRO, DANCE AND COMPETITIONS

# There's more to ballet than buns and tutus

A good acrobat can make tricks look beautiful by straightening their legs and pointing their toes—the foundations of ballet. In ballet, you're constantly stretching your knees and feet in all exercises (at the barre and in the centre), which strengthens muscles and improves technique. This helps you learn how to activate the muscles in your legs and feet in a very specific way. You also perfect your arm lines and learn how to move your hands in a beautiful way. On top of that, you build a lot of strength in your legs, which helps in acro as well as loads of other styles.

All of this adds up to make ballet the ultimate all-round improver: good technique in this discipline makes your dancing more elegant and precise, no matter which genre of dance you're trying to learn (except, maybe, hip-hop).

When we watch kids do acro, we can always spot the ones who do ballet because they have more control, which is also hugely important in acro. Now that we are ballet teachers ourselves, we love it when there are acro students in our ballet classes because we know how much they're going to improve. We always tell them, 'This is going to help your acro so much.'

Years ago, people didn't think ballet and acro mixed. Ballet is all about keeping a straight back, while acro is the opposite. But now, acro teachers see the benefits of doing ballet, and these days, being a well-rounded, versatile dancer is highly encouraged. Even though people are naturally better at certain styles of dance, being able to do many styles well means you'll be a better and more employable dancer, if you're looking to make it a career.

Teagan is more of a 'pretty' dancer, so she leans towards ballet and lyrical dance, whereas Sam prefers harder-hitting styles such as hip-hop and jazz. But obviously, we both want to be as good as we can be at all genres, so we have taken classes in all of them.

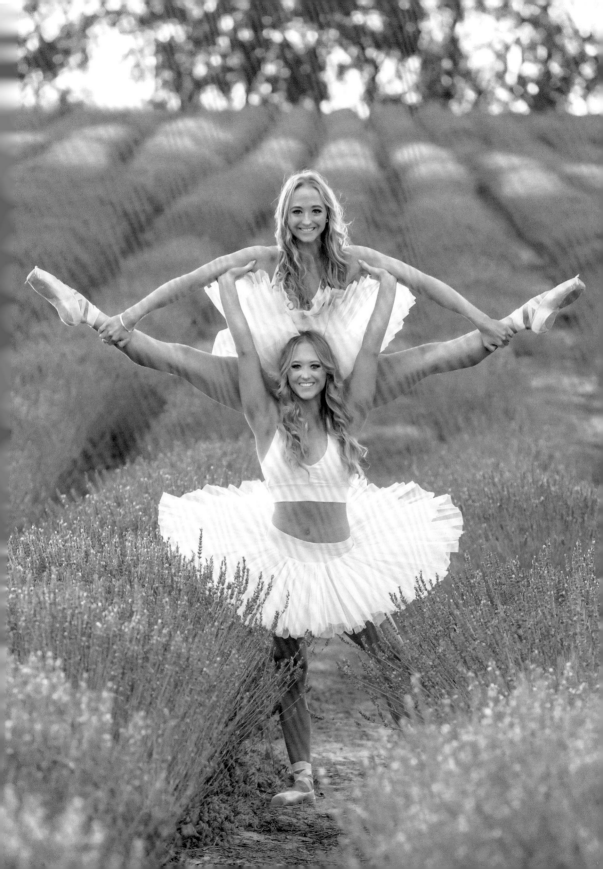

If we're practising a combo that includes a style of dance one of us is naturally better at, the twin who isn't quite as good will get inspired by watching the way the other one does certain movements. For example, Teagan might watch how Sam hits certain hip-hop moves, then try to copy them so they look just as good when she does them. We don't want our individual preferences to affect how we look when we dance—and we enjoy the challenge of dancing all of the styles, anyway.

## Trust us: ballet will make you better!

When we were younger, whenever we'd see a girl who was amazing at dancing, we'd get so inspired. We'd ask Mum, 'Why is she so good?' and she would say, 'It's because she does a lot of ballet.' Naturally, it wasn't long before we wanted to do extra ballet lessons. Some people don't find ballet the most fun (let's be honest, some people find it boring), but we had a reason for doing it: it would take our dance and acro to the next level.

A note from ... *Sam*

When it came to us doing extra ballet classes to improve as acrobats and dancers, Teagan was totally happy to do that because she'd always loved ballet. I was a little slower to come around to the idea. I'd always felt I wasn't very good at ballet, and because of that, I didn't really like it. So, the first year that Teagan enrolled in the extra ballet class, I decided to give it a miss.

By the end of the year, I noticed that Teagan had improved a lot, and she was ranking higher than me at competitions. Even though I was working as hard as her, and practising just as much, I wasn't as good. I'd think, 'Okay, what is it? Do I need to stretch my legs more? Improve my leaps? Show my personality more?'

Whenever I competed against anyone better than me, including Teagan, those dancers would inspire me and become my motivation to improve. I'm a very competitive person when it comes to dancing or sports, and, like Teagan, I always strive to be the best that I can be at whatever I'm doing. When I asked myself what Teagan was doing that I wasn't, there was only one answer: ballet.

When enrolment time came around the next year, I said to Mum, 'Do you think I should do that extra ballet class?' As usual, she said it was up to me.

After a minute, I said, 'Yeah, I'm going to do it this year, too.' And I did, only this time it felt different. This time, I knew why I was doing it. I had seen what a difference ballet could make, and that pushed me to put so much more effort into every class. As my focus improved, my ballet technique improved, too. Once that happened, I started loving ballet. And I soon saw the same improvements that Teagan had.

If I hadn't pushed myself to take those extra classes, I would have missed out on something I now love so much. I'm glad I stuck with it. Sometimes, the things we find the hardest are the things that are the most worth doing.

95

We now teach ballet to eight-, nine- and ten-year-olds, and because we know how important ballet is, we're passionate teachers. We want our kids to love it for the same reasons we do. One of the very first things we say to our students (and something we remind them of throughout the year) is that if they put their best effort into the class, they will improve. If you're bored in ballet, you aren't working hard enough. Being bored means you aren't listening or applying the techniques properly.

When we see someone yawning in class, or not listening, it's frustrating, because we want to see our students get better and succeed. We know the information we are sharing can really help them, but only if they are willing to put in the work. If we see kids playing around, we try to guide them and get them back on track by reminding them of the end goal. We'll say, 'You're the one who wants to improve, right? That's why you're here, isn't it?' But we also make sure we incorporate a little fun with ballet games, so it's not all serious, all the time.

If you've tried ballet before and given up, or if you're in ballet right now and not loving it, just know that you'll get so much more satisfaction and enjoyment from it when your technique and strength improves, and you're able to do ballet well. But it isn't an overnight thing; you must work your way up there first. It's worth it, though. We can pretty much guarantee that if you work hard enough to see the results, you'll start to love it. You must try your absolute best for that hour if you want to reap the rewards.

## Comp life prepares you for real life

When we think of ourselves as dancers, it almost feels as though our lives have been all about comps—in a good way! We were always thinking about the next one, training, working on getting better, making or not making it into the championships. Being involved in competitions from a young age helped us improve so much as dancers by giving us concrete goals to work towards.

Every school holiday, we'd be in full-on competition mode. This process taught us so much about life and gave us many valuable skills. We even learned how to do our own hair and make-up at comps, back in the days before YouTube tutorials!

Dance comps are like their own world. They've got their own traditions, etiquette, language and style. Being away and competing, surrounded by so many great dancers and friends, was always the best experience.

We feel so lucky that we've been able to not only compete in lots of big comps, but also to win prizes that allowed us to travel and have incredible experiences. Many of the dance comps in Australia offer amazing prizes, such as a trip to the United States to compete in competitions there. Winning certain comps in Australia allows you to take classes at prestigious dance schools in cities such as London and Los Angeles. Comps opened so many doors for us. In Australia, there used to be only a few competitions each year. Now, there are so many to choose from, just like the United States. From when we were very young, Mum would take us to comps to watch older dancers compete. We absolutely loved it, and aspired to be like those older girls. By the time we were nine, we had decided that we were ready to enter our first acro competition. Both of us were a little too nervous to do a solo for our very first competition, so we entered as a duo. It was still scary, but at least we'd have each other.

That year, there weren't many people in our section, so the organisers expanded the group to include ages nine to twelve. Not only were we competing for the very first time, but also now we were going up against much older girls!

We were so motivated to practise and push ourselves because it was our first time competing and this was a big deal for us. Every single day after school, without fail, we practised. The coaching we got from Mum and Miss Deb was crucial in helping us develop our discipline of regular practise. Without their encouragement, we wouldn't have been able to improve as much or get our routine to the level we did.

Our family's lounge room was one of our favourite spots to practise. We couldn't do the routines full-out, but we'd get all the choreography right and then, once we were ready, we'd try the routine in a bigger place—usually the local oval.

## The first of many comps

Your first competition can be daunting, and at nine, we were both scared to get on that stage. The idea of going out there in front of everyone, trying to get everything in the routine correct and be up against other people was … terrifying!

In the dressing room before we went on, Sam started crying and saying that she didn't think she could do it. Mum was trying to calm us down (without much success) when two senior girls from our dance school, Tash and Ciaira, came over and said to Mum, 'Don't worry, leave them with us.' So, Mum went and sat down in the audience and left us with them, and they took over.

This was all a long time ago, so we don't remember exactly what they said to us backstage, we just remember really liking that they were there for us. They were older than us, so they were the girls we looked up to, and it felt so nice to have their support.

Whatever they said or did must have worked, because

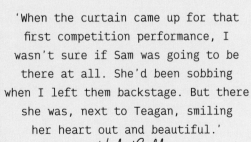

'When the curtain came up for that first competition performance, I wasn't sure if Sam was going to be there at all. She'd been sobbing when I left them backstage. But there she was, next to Teagan, smiling her heart out and beautiful.'
— Vicki Rybka

we managed to not only get on stage, but also control our nerves. And the rush of getting out there and performing our first routine was incredible. All that practising paid off, and we ended up coming second in our section.

A note from ... *Teagan*

Ever since that very first competition, Sam and I have always competed as an acro duo. But the next year, I decided I also wanted to compete with an acro solo. I don't really remember why; I probably just wanted to test myself, to see if I could do it.

So, at ten, I competed with my solo, and—gotta be honest—it didn't go very well! I got out of time with the music, and was off on my personality because I was thinking about the choreography and what I was doing. Basically, I let nerves get the better of me. Needless to say, I didn't get anywhere in that comp. It was a big section that year, and I was nowhere near making the cut.

Sometimes, it's just not your day. Sometimes you get scared or forget your moves—especially when you're young. That is why competitions are so good for young performers and athletes: they teach you how to conquer those nerves and help you improve for the next one. You can't go out there thinking that you're going to be amazing the first (or even second) time you compete. Work towards that, but remember, it takes time.

# Make friends with your fear

So many people ask us if we still get nervous before we perform. Ummm ... YES! Every. Single. Time.

Putting yourself out there—whether you're dancing, singing in front of a bunch of people or giving a speech—can be terrifying. Even though we've been doing this for so long, we still get nervous before everything we do. The fact is, when you really care about something, getting nervous about it is just part of the deal.

If you want to succeed, though, it's important to learn to stay on top of those nerves as much as you can. Find something that works for you, whether that's listening to music, taking a few deep breaths or distracting yourself in some way. Although nerves are completely normal, if you let your thoughts run out of control, it might mean you get a bit shaky when you perform and then aren't able to stick your tricks as well. You must find that happy medium and a way to handle your fears.

Nerves don't have to be bad though; you can even use them to your advantage. The extra adrenaline pumping through you right before you step on stage can give you the energy to jump higher or give a trick that extra effort. By the time the music starts, you should have practised so much that you're 100 per cent confident in what you're doing. It's almost as if your body should be able to move on autopilot—it's time to just perform and enjoy.

When we perform, it's almost as if we're playing the character of that dance or song; we're not ourselves. People who've seen us perform often say we look so confident (even when we don't feel that way), and they're surprised to find out that we're pretty shy when we first meet people.

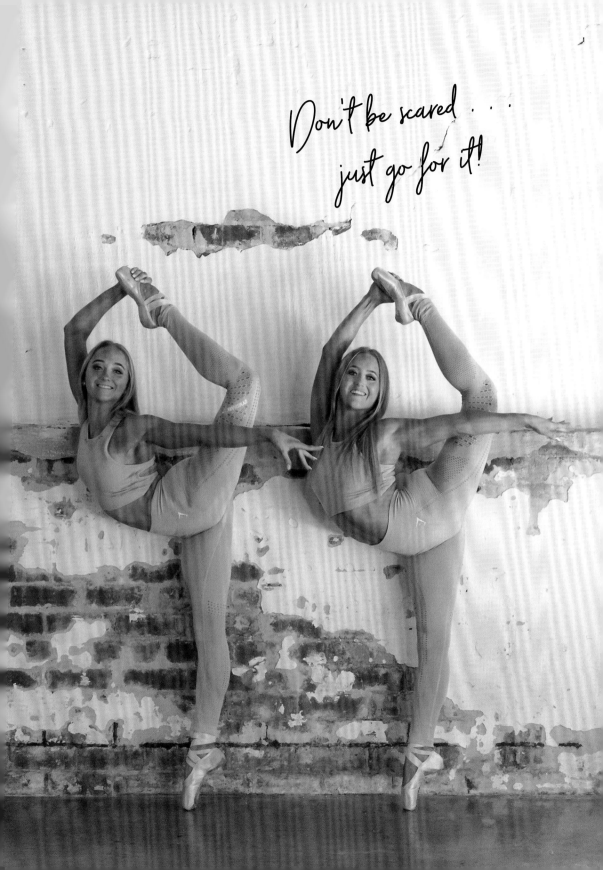

Don't be scared . . .
just go for it!

# HARD WORK BEATS TALENT

# WHEN TALENT DOESN'T

*Work Hard*

— Tim Notke

# Set big goals

Another saying both of us love is from Tim Notke and it goes, 'Hard work beats talent when talent doesn't work hard.' This sentiment is spot on. It doesn't matter how naturally talented someone is at something—if someone else is willing to put in more time and effort, the hard worker is going to come out on top. Practice makes perfect.

We have practised a lot. Every school holiday we'd spend many days at acro or dance classes, or preparing routines for a comp. If we weren't at class, we were working on things at home. Practising became second nature, and it got to the point where, if we were out somewhere and saw good grass, we'd be like, 'Ooh, that looks really good to tumble on,' and off we'd go.

## Park life

We've always loved practising outside on grass, and we still love being outside and doing our routines at parks. People often stop and watch us or beep their horns as they drive by. Looking the same makes us distinctive, so we're known as those twins who do acro at the park or oval. One time, when we were working at the McDonald's drive-through, a customer even asked, 'Are you the twins who are always down at the park?' We just laughed and nodded.

When we were quite young, we noticed that in some sections, the winner would win a huge trophy as well as the standard-size trophy. This big trophy is known as the 'perpetual trophy'. Of course, our first question was, 'How do we win that big one?' Mum explained that, in order to win it, we'd have to win in the open category, which includes all the dancers who've come first in the novice section of that age group and genre in previous competitions.

It wasn't long before winning this big trophy became our ultimate goal. Teagan won her first perpetual trophies when she was eleven for her acro and jazz solos, and Sam won hers when she was seventeen for an acro solo—such an exciting day. Winning those trophies made us feel our hard work was paying off. It's not just about winning but working towards something: no matter what stage of life you are in, it's important to have goals.

In 2015, we won a comp in Australia, and the prize was a trip to the United States, to attend a competition in Seattle. This was our first time competing in the US, and it was such an exciting opportunity.

We flew to Seattle with a team of dancers, but on the day of the comp, we were so jet-lagged that we were struggling! As we'd come all the way from Australia, the competition organisers wanted to livestream our performance so our friends and family back home could watch (how nice is that?). But unfortunately, the tech kept failing so our performance kept getting pushed back. We kept warming up so we'd be ready when they needed us, but eventually we had to lie down because we were just so tired. We so wanted to sleep, but then we were like, nah, we've come all this way. We have to do it!

Acro is one of the most physically demanding dance styles, so you must be mentally ready before a performance. Before we went on, we had to rev each other up so we could get in the right headspace and keep our energy levels up. Our duo performance went really well, and we ended up getting the highest score out of that whole comp. The judges and the audience gave us a standing ovation—people were going crazy! We'll never forget it.

## So, you want a career in dance?

If you love dance with a passion and work really hard, there are many career possibilities out there that you may not have even thought about. When you're young, it's impossible to know what's going to happen in your future. We always knew we wanted to do something with dancing; we just weren't sure what that would be.

When we were doing all those classes, we didn't realise that this hobby we loved so much would turn into a career.

Thankfully, all the training when we were young set us up for the life we live now. All the money our parents spent on lessons, competitions and costumes, and all those hours we spent practising and going to classes, wasn't wasted. When you get to do a job that you've worked towards all your life, you can share your passion in a way that feels true to who you are. A lot of young dancers think there's just one career out there: back-up dancer. But when you start digging a little more, you realise that's only the tip of the iceberg.

Besides our YouTube channel, both of us teach dance classes for different dance styles and age groups. Sometimes, we also perform at events or on dance tours, and that's always exciting. We also have a Bachelor of Education, which means we're qualified to teach dance and drama at a secondary-education level.

A note from ... *Sam*

I know this is going to sound crazy, but whenever I get a payment for teaching dance or performing at an event, I've almost forgotten that I was going to be paid for it. I'll see the payment and say to myself, 'Oh yeah, this is a job!'

It's not that money isn't important to me, or that I don't need to be paid for my work, it's just that it's second nature for us to teach a class or perform. In our minds, we're doing the same things we've always done—only now, people are paying us! Don't get us wrong: it's hard work. But it's what we've always done, and it's genuinely so fun that being paid feels like a bonus.

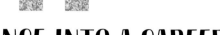

# TURNING DANCE INTO A CAREER

If you love dance like we do but aren't sure how to make a career from it, here are a few ideas:

- 🤍 You can **teach** (like we do!), either at a school, teaching casual dance classes, or at a dance studio. You could even open your own dance studio. There are so many types of dance schools out there; you could have a cheerleading school, an acro school, a dedicated ballet school or a school that offers all genres.
- 🤍 You could be a **performer** in Cirque du Soleil.
- 🤍 You could be a **choreographer**. There are so many different roles for a choreographer—you could do this for music videos, shows, big events, theatre . . . the list goes on!
- 🤍 If you love being around the world of dance, you could go into **lighting, set design, costume or make-up**.
- 🤍 You could be a **dance physiotherapist**. One of our friends is a physio and a former dancer. She's able to relate really well to patients who are dancers because she understands the exact tricks and moves they are asking about, and can be specific about what they can and can't do while recovering from their injury.
- 🤍 Dance is good preparation for **modelling**. One of our dance friends models now, and she brings that dancer's edge to being a great model, because she holds herself beautifully and comes up with creative poses (yass Nikita!).

- You could be a **performer** at a theme park or on a cruise ship. This can be a fun job, but it can also be tough to get work because you may need to fit a specific character description. For example, if you're auditioning at Disneyland, you might be the most amazing dancer but if you don't have a 'Cinderella' look, you may miss out. That's just how it goes. We have a friend whose dream was to be a princess at Disneyland. After auditions and rejections, she's finally off to Disneyland Paris and to live her dream. We are so happy for her. It proves you should never give up on your dream. (Congrats, Ash!)
- You could work as a **back-up dancer** for pop stars. This is probably the career that sounds most exciting to most dancers, but it's insanely competitive. A lot of successful singers are based in the United States, so that's where most of the work is. You have to be very lucky to make it as a back-up dancer, because there's so much competition, but don't let this stop you. If this is your dream, go for it. As with the theme parks, it's not always down to how well you dance. People casting a tour or a video will usually have a specific 'look' they're aiming for, so again, you must be an amazing dancer and happen to have that look. You never know, this could be you.
- You can be a **dancer in theatre productions**, such as Broadway shows, or be a dancer in a company.
- You can start your own **social media** career, for example on Instagram or YouTube, and share your passion and hard work with people from all around the world (like we do!).

If you want to make dance a career, the earlier you start, the better. But no matter when you start, or what your particular talents are, do whatever you can to make your dream a reality.

## A note about posting on social media

If you are under eighteen years old, never post on YouTube, Instagram or any other social media without first getting your parents' approval. This is important. The internet is a great place for sharing, but only if an adult is aware of what you're doing. And if you ever feel threatened, unsafe or in any way uncomfortable about how someone is talking to you online, tell a parent, teacher or other adult right away. (We'll go into more detail about this in Chapter 8.)

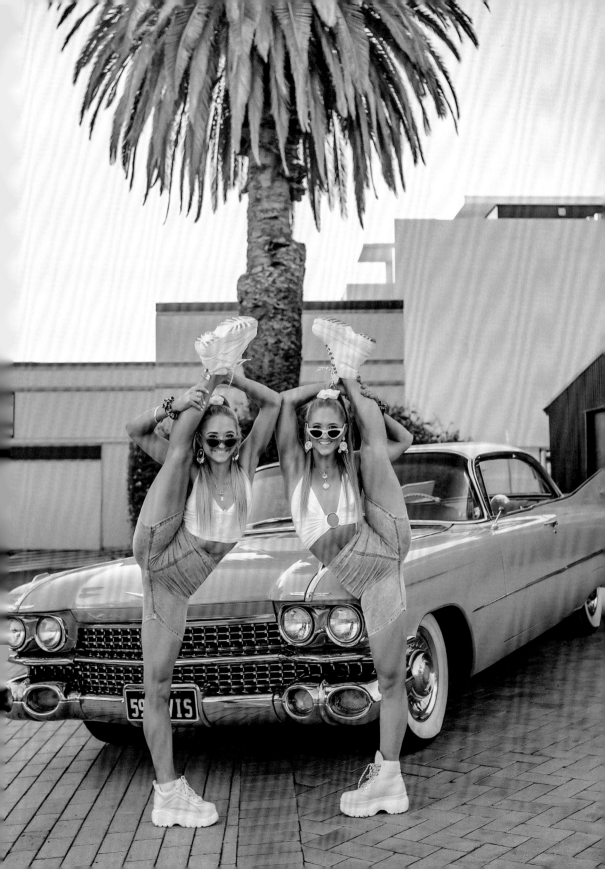

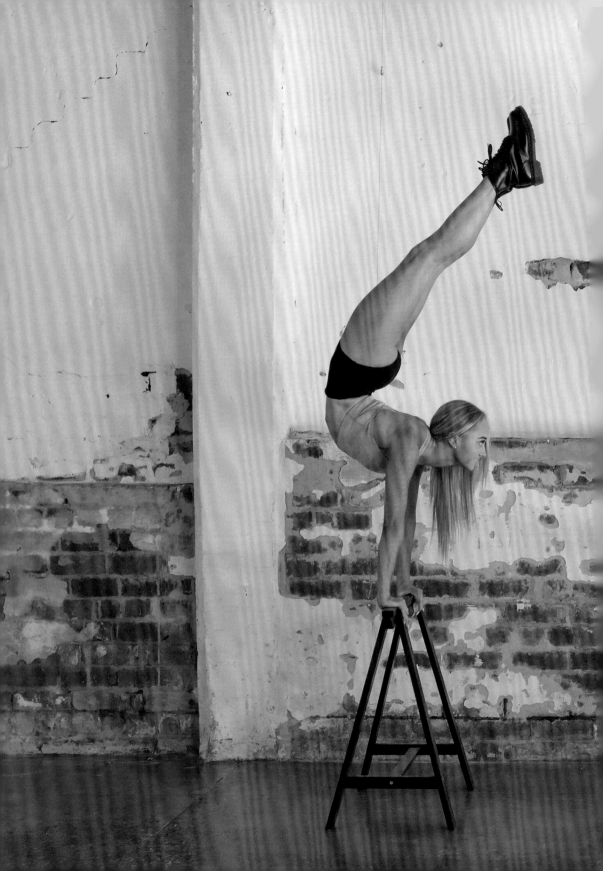

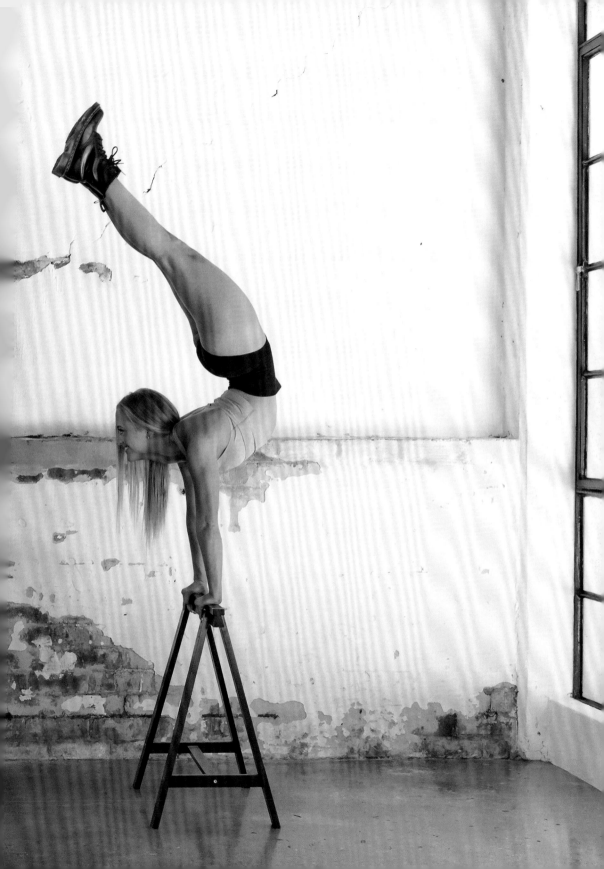

# CHAPTER 5

# Firm, fun AND fair!

F irm, fun and fair: these four words sum up our teaching style perfectly! It's what we want from a teacher when we're in a class, and it's what we try to be now that we're teachers. We mostly teach classes together because we love it and work well together as a team, but we also teach on our own, too.

Our university degrees taught us a lot, but many of the skills and approaches we use with those we teach now come from our experiences of being students for so many years.

We are definitely a little strict, and we expect a lot from our students. We like to set clear expectations from the start of each term. For example, ballet dancers must wear stockings, leotards and ballet shoes to classes, and their hair must be in a tidy bun. We always say that if you want to dance, you must wear the uniform of a dancer. If a police officer were to rock up to work in her pyjamas, would you have the same level of respect for her? Would you even know she was a police officer? Our students get it, and right from their very first class with us, they know to show up looking like proper ballerinas.

Another thing that's important to us is that our students are respectful. Unfortunately, we occasionally encounter students who don't show respect—they'll come in late or they won't listen to instructions. We were always taught that if you come late to class, it's important to acknowledge your teacher, or at least smile. We'll pick our kids up on things like this, too.

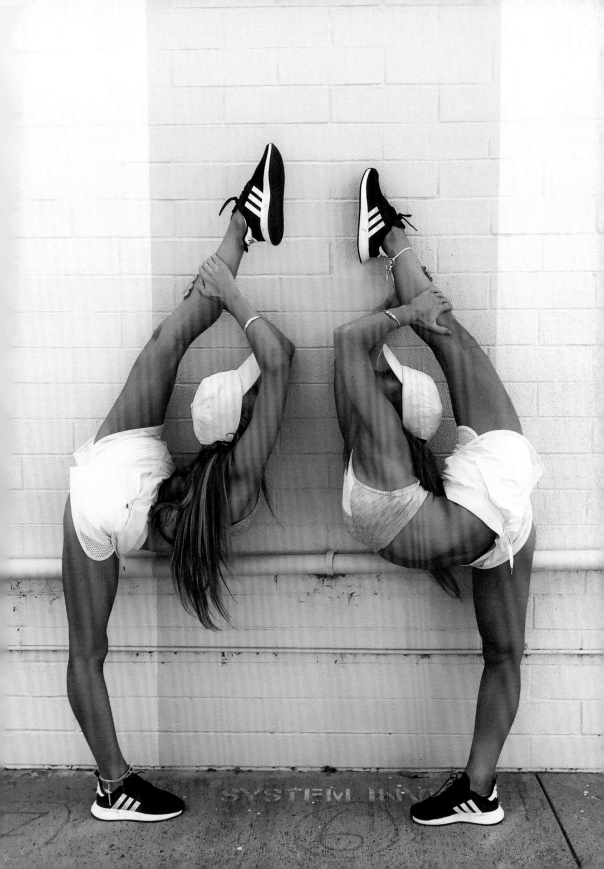

As a teacher, it's important to recognise and accept everyone in the room, not just the loud kids in the front row. Each term, we make an effort to learn everyone's names and get to know and understand the different personalities. We also try to make time to connect at the beginning of each class; we'll ask what everyone has been up to that week. You can break down a lot of walls this way. Every now and then, at the end of class, we leave time to play a fun dance-related game, so class ends on a high.

The years we've put into dance, and the experiences we've had, have given us so much knowledge to share with our students. And because we know how many amazing (and fun) opportunities can come from being a good dancer, we are passionate teachers. A teacher creates the vibe in the room; a good teacher can make class fun and inspire you at the same time.

*Trust* that whatever the teacher has to say will make you a *better dancer* in some way.

• • •

We approach the classes we attend as students with the understanding that every teacher has something to offer. If we stay open, we're always going to learn something. It might only be one thing, but that one thing might be valuable in the future. Even bad teachers can teach you something (like what not to do in the future). So, whenever you walk into a class, assume that you'll learn something and trust that whatever the teacher has to say will make you a better dancer in some way.

We've had a lot of great teachers, and we're so grateful for them because they've each given us something and made us the dancers we are today. Naturally, everyone has a favourite teacher or two, and as we've gotten older, the teachers we've formed strong connections with are also considered friends. Being friends with your teachers isn't necessarily encouraged, but because we are older, this naturally happens sometimes.

We love teachers who don't bring their mood to dance class, something we try to mirror in our own teaching style. No matter what's going on in their personal lives, they remain professional and show up to every class vibrant, happy and ready to do their job.

Another thing a good teacher can do is explain their corrections. Sometimes, corrections will get thrown at you and you may not understand what the teacher means, or how to fix whatever it is you're doing. A good teacher will be able to come up with clear metaphors and explanations to help you picture exactly what you're doing wrong. This way, you'll understand what needs to be done and can use the critique they've given you to improve. The metaphors and explanations we've heard over the years have stuck with us, and we're able to remember them. Now that we are teachers, we try to teach our students the same way.

## Criticism is not a bad thing

We know, especially after completing our teaching degrees, that it's not really 'done' these days to single out students in class to criticise something they are doing. But in the dance world, this kind of thing isn't only accepted, it's necessary. Critiques are a key part of dancing. Learning how to take criticism well and use it to your advantage can help you develop a thicker skin, which is a valuable asset in life outside of dance.

Nobody likes being told they are doing something wrong, but the fact is, when it comes to certain things, there is a right way and a wrong way to do them. Dancers get critiqued a lot, but when a teacher is hard on you, it's usually because they want you to reach your full potential. If we're doing something wrong, we want to know what it is so we can fix it.

Sometimes, other parents would complain to Mum about certain teachers that Mum knew were fully qualified. They'd tell her that the teacher was picking on their daughter by correcting her all the time, and Mum would say, 'She's so lucky that the teacher is paying attention to her. She's trying to make her a better dancer.'

Mum has always been firm and straight with us. She tells it like it is. She's not going to give us praise if we haven't earned it, so when she says we've done a great job, we know she means it. Sometimes the truth can hurt, but we'd rather know where we stand.

In our opinion, not getting honest feedback just sets you up for a fall. Eventually, someone is going to tell you the truth, and if you aren't expecting criticism, the honesty will sting that much more. Even worse, if you have a false sense of your talent, you might not even believe the criticism or take it on board. We believe it's better to be real with someone so they can take the opportunity to improve if they need to.

*Believe us, you want all the corrections.*

• • •

Of course, it feels a little embarrassing to be singled out in a class and corrected, but if you can get past that, listen to what you're being told and apply the advice you've just been given, it's for the best—it will help you. Believe us, you want all the corrections. It means a teacher is watching you, cares about you and wants you to get better. If you aren't getting critiqued, you're being left behind. Even when we're teaching kids that we know are just in dance class for fun, we'll still encourage them to do things properly because we want them to improve. Doing something for fun doesn't mean you can't be amazing at the level you are at.

So, the next time a teacher tells you your arm is in the wrong spot, remember that they're doing it to help you. Take a deep breath, listen to the correction, and then try to use it to get better.

118

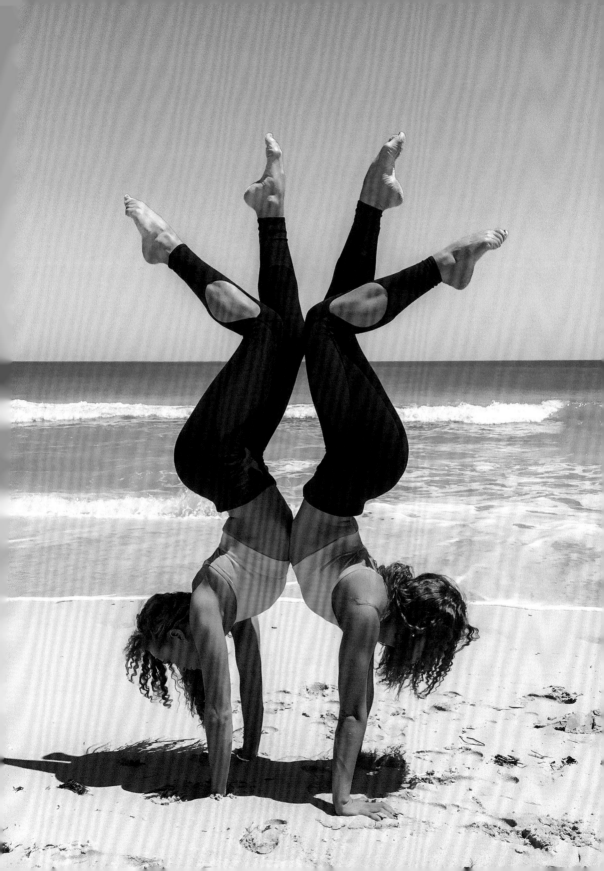

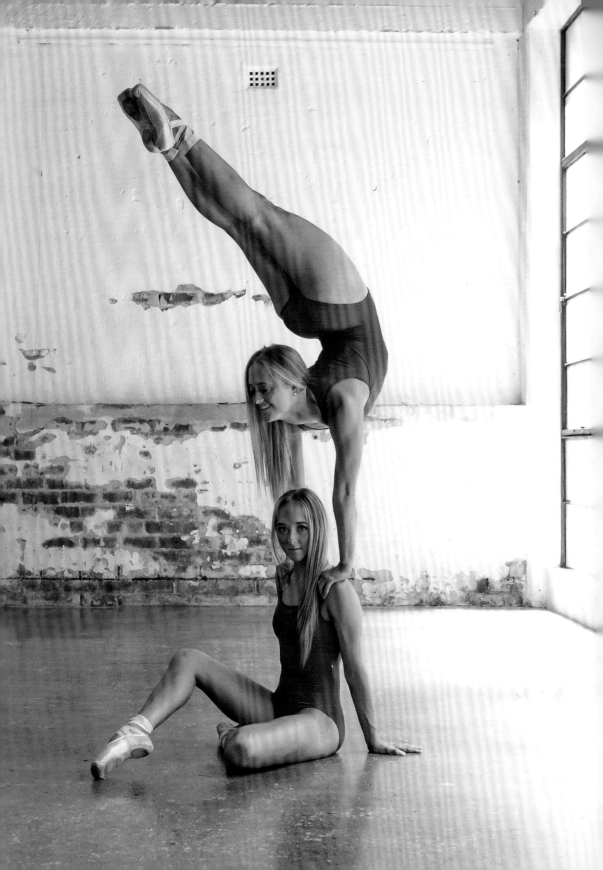

# Toughen up, buttercup!

When we were young, one of our first dance teachers was very strict. Not in a scary way, but we knew we couldn't muck around in her class. She taught us to respect our teachers. She was passionate about dancing, and any beginners in her class got a great start. Some kids used to say she was a bit mean, and it was only when we grew up that we realised she was actually the nicest lady. She just wanted the best results from us, and to make sure we knew what we were doing. (Thanks Miss Bev!)

Even today, both of us prefer teachers who are tough on us. (Are we crazy or what?) This probably reflects our upbringing: Mum and Dad were great parents. They always pushed us, and we liked that. Mum was brought up with very strict dance teachers—way more so than today. Times have changed!

We were brought up to be resilient and not make a big deal about little things. As teachers, we know there are some things that genuinely stop a student from attending class, or affect what they can do. But if the problem a student is complaining about isn't a real issue, we like to encourage them to push on.

This is Miss Nicki ... one of our amazing teachers who taught us for many years and got us through all of our major ballet exams!

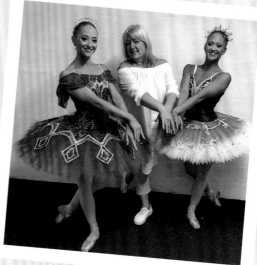

# Dealing with physical setbacks

When you play sports or do physical activities, it's normal to face challenges with your body, either with injuries or illnesses. These times can be hard. Not being able to do the thing you love can seem unfair and make you feel down.

We've had our share of challenges, from broken bones and gastro to migraines during competitions. The way we've dealt with these setbacks is to focus on what we can do, not what we can't. Injuries aren't permanent (most of the time), and if you have a good doctor and are following their advice, you should be able to get back to full power once you recover. If an injury means you'll be out for weeks or months, there are probably ways you can keep the rest of your body strong. When your body is used to activity, you can lose muscle tone quickly once you stop, and you don't want that to happen if you can avoid it. Don't let a small setback turn into a bigger one.

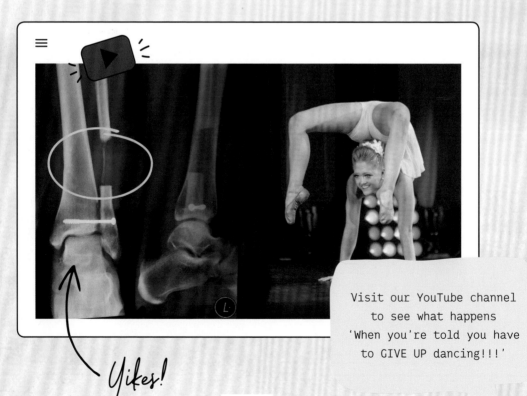

*Yikes!*

Visit our YouTube channel to see what happens 'When you're told you have to GIVE UP dancing!!!'

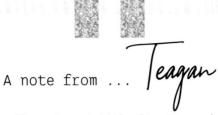

A note from ... *Teagan*

When I was fifteen, I was told I had to give up dancing. Sam and I had been mucking around on the grass doing a whole heap of acro, especially one trick we were trying again and again: a no-handed somersault in the air to land on your feet. We really wanted to get it, so every day for about a week or two, we'd come home from school and practise that move. Eventually, we got it. And once we did, we did it multiple times.

While we were doing this trick, I started noticing a pain in my leg. I ignored it for a couple weeks, but it wasn't going away so I told Mum. She took me to get checked out and have an X-ray. When the doctor came back with the results, he told Mum there was a tumour or a lesion on my leg. It turned out to be a lesion, and the doctor said that for it to break down and heal, I was going to have to stop dancing completely because dancing would put too much pressure on the lesion.

I was devastated! Mum decided to get a second opinion, and she found a great sports injury specialist. He said that he didn't think that I needed to give up dancing completely, but that I would need to take it a bit easy, that it was going to hurt if I danced and might even get worse. He also said that if it started hurting, I had to rest it and not go full out.

To be honest, I probably pushed myself harder than I should have. I kept doing everything as normal. I put up with the pain when I danced, but eventually it got so bad that I was unable to do lots of moves. So, we went back to the doctor to get an update and find out if my lesion had shrunk.

The next X-ray showed that instead of breaking down as expected, my lesion had doubled in size! The doctor diagnosed it as an aneurysmal bone cyst, which was going to keep growing. He said they'd have to remove it. This would be the first surgery I'd ever had, so I was freaking out. The plan was for them to go in and scrape the cyst out of my bone, and the recovery time was going to be pretty long. We tried to figure out the best time of year for the surgery, when the recovery time would least affect comps and other things I had going on. I didn't want to miss out on anything.

On the day of the surgery, about five minutes before I was due to go into the operating theatre, the specialist came in to tell us that he'd been doing some last-minute research about the procedure and had decided to do something different. He wasn't going to scrape it out after all; he was going to go in and take that part of bone out completely. And this was going to involve a much longer recovery period as my bone grew back. Great!

He said I'd be walking within three months, and fully recovered after twelve. I was in complete shock, but he believed it would give me the best chance of a full recovery, so we went for it.

After the surgery, I was on crutches for two months. At the beginning, just the pain of putting any pressure on my leg was so bad it was hard to imagine I'd ever be able to do flips or leaps. After about three months, I got a moonboot. I cried the day I got my moonboot because I was so embarrassed about having to wear it! But, once I got used to moving around with it, I focused on keeping the rest of my body strong and flexible. I'd do tricks and push-ups that didn't involve my bad leg.

If you have an injury, it's important to talk to a good sports doctor or physio to make sure you never do anything that puts you at risk or makes your condition worse. But you will also probably find that you don't need to stop doing everything, either. Your muscles can weaken quickly when they aren't used, so try to do what you can.

During that year, I did everything I could to stay strong and keep myself in good shape, even though the leg I'd had surgery on was definitely weaker. You could look at it and see that it was skinnier than my other leg. But I wanted to be part of my dance studio's end-of-year performance, so I was working towards that. That was my goal. I felt that if I could be on stage with my friends and do most things, I'd be happy with that.

It took a whole year for my strength to get back to normal. This was a scary time in my life. I got upset and frustrated, but I also worked hard to catch up and be an even better dancer than I was before. In a way, I'm even grateful for this experience now. It taught me not to give up, even when things seem impossible.

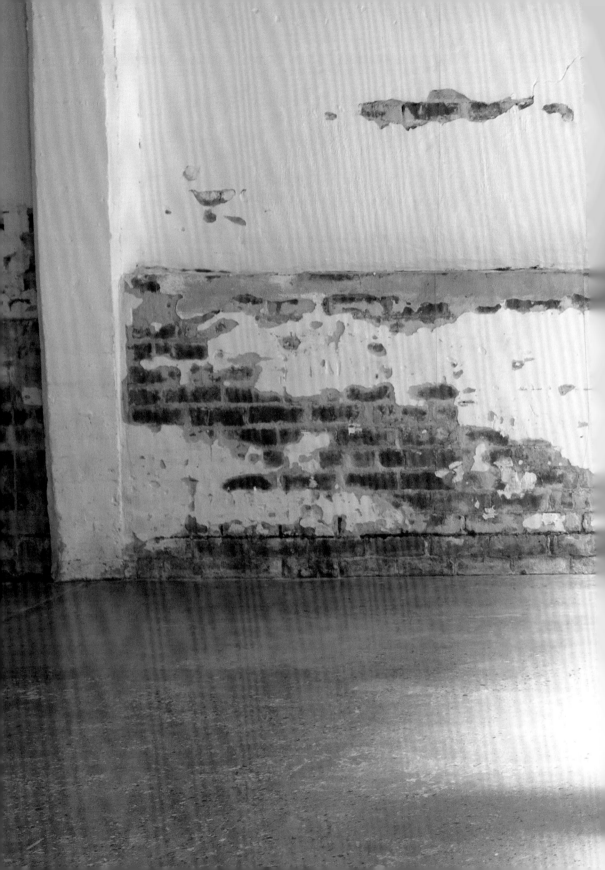

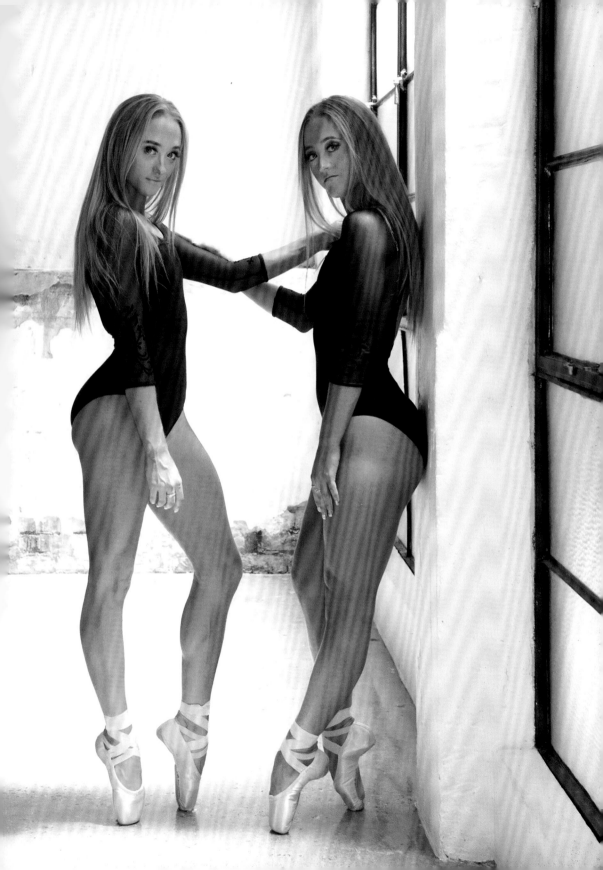

# The lighter side of dance

During the first half of the school year, most of what goes on in dance class is based on exam work (though not all dance schools focus on this), whereas the second half of year is more relaxed because you're working on routines for the end-of-year concert. Working towards any performance is always fun for us. It's great for motivation, too. It doesn't matter what that performance is for, just knowing you will perform in front of people means you're a more focused dancer. And even if you're only taking dance for fun or exercise, rather than to compete, getting ready for the concert is still exciting because you're showcasing everything you've been practising throughout the year, and getting up on a stage.

End-of-year concerts always meant so much to us, especially when we were younger. You get to perform in full costume on a real stage, and friends and family can see what you've been working hard at all year—plus, you get to do it with all of your friends.

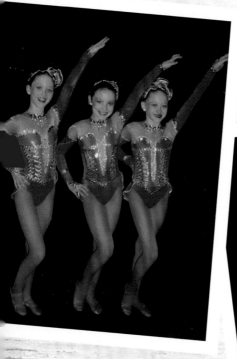

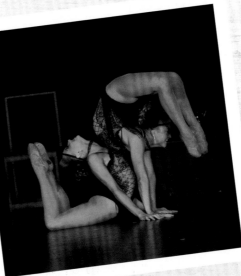

We've had the pleasure of performing at numerous end-of-year dance concerts.

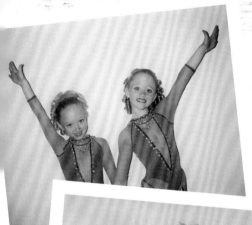

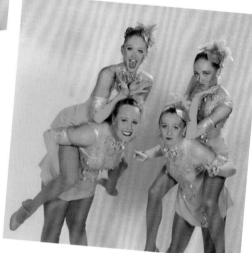

*It's showtime!*

# CHOOSING A DANCE SCHOOL THAT SUITS *you*

When our first dance school shut down, Mum had to find a new school to send us to. If there are lots of dance schools in your area, this can be daunting—especially if you don't know much about dance. A good tip for parents is to pick a school you're interested in and either go and watch their end-of-year concert or ask to borrow a DVD of it from the school. Concerts can be a good way to get a sense of the quality of teaching and feel of a place.

Another good tip is to book a trial class at a few different schools and see which one vibes best. Depending on how often you'll be going to the studio, it might be a good idea to choose a school reasonably close to home or school, though if you're more serious about dance, it can be worth travelling to a better school farther away.

# CHAPTER 6

# Australia's got Talent

In 2008, when we were twelve years old, one of Mum's friends mentioned this new TV show, *Australia's Got Talent*. We hadn't heard of it at that point. She told us they were going to be holding auditions around the country for the second series, and suggested we try out for it when they came to Perth. Not really knowing much about it, we said, 'Yeah, okay. We could give that a go.' Now, thinking back, we can't believe we had the courage to do it. We were young and so much shyer than we are today.

When the open audition day came around, we went along to an auditorium, along with hundreds of other acts, and didn't really know what to expect. The way it works on the show is that performers pre-audition for the TV producers, who then decide whether they can go on to the next round a few months later, which is the live TV audition in front of an audience and celebrity judges.

We auditioned with a Russian-themed routine that we'd used for a competition. Although the producers liked us, there were Cossack dancers in the show already. They asked if we had other routines we could do, and of course we said yes. After that first audition, we ended up choreographing another two routines—one to 'Mambo No Five', and a can-can routine. The producers chose the can-can, and said they were happy for us to use that one for our TV audition.

There were a few months between that very first audition and our live TV audition, so we had some time to perfect our

new routine, and we needed it more than we probably realised!
As part of our rehearsal process, Mum used to film us doing our
routines so we could watch them back and fix any issues. We've still
got footage of us practising that routine, and when we watch those
videos now, they are laughable! The routine was so terrible when we
started; we were out of time, not pointing our toes, our legs weren't
near our heads. You can hear Mum in the background shouting
corrections at us (in a nice way, LOL!). Basically, we were so bad.

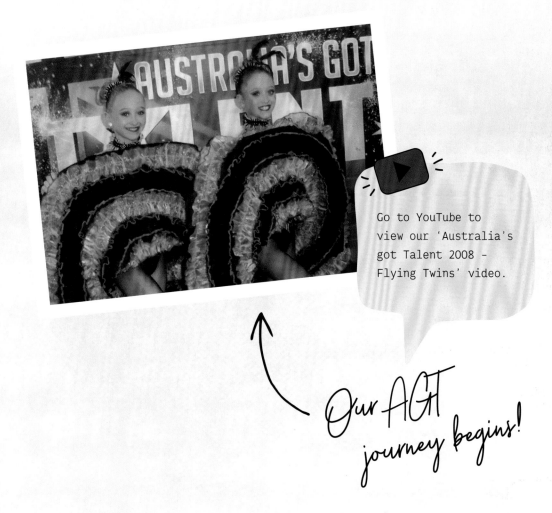

Go to YouTube to
view our 'Australia's
got Talent 2008 -
Flying Twins' video.

*Our AGT journey begins!*

133

We'd come home from school every day, change clothes and go straight to the oval to work on the routine. We kept changing the choreography, too, to make it better. Eventually, after all that practice time, we got the routine to a level worthy of being on TV. When we compare the polished routine that was shown on TV to the beginning of our rehearsal process, it's night and day! We can't believe how far we managed to come in that short space of time.

Getting the chance to audition for the celebrity judges on TV was a big deal for us. That year, the judges were Dannii Minogue, Tom Burlinson and Red Symons. The filmed audition is a bit of a blur for us now; we just remember feeling so shy, but also excited about getting to showcase our dancing. We wanted people to see what we'd been practising so hard for.

Back then, our stage name was 'Double Impact'. On the day of the live taping in Melbourne, our performance went well and our hard work paid off. The three celebrity judges liked us, although Dannii Minogue didn't feel comfortable that we'd lifted up our can-can skirts during the performance. She thought it was a little inappropriate. She said 'yes' to putting us through to the next round but asked us to wear something different next time. We were so confused. What else would you wear for a can-can routine besides a can-can costume?

When we watched that TV performance later, we realised that the music was different. It turned out that the music we'd danced to hadn't been cleared for use on TV, so they'd ended up having to dub in different music when it aired. It was pretty seamless, so whoever did the audio did a great job.

We were on top of the world after that performance, but, as we soon found out, in TV world, getting three yesses doesn't guarantee you will go through to the next round. The producers explained that there were too many acts potentially going through, so they'd have to call and let us know. When we didn't end up making it any further, we were crushed. But even so, we still felt good about what we had accomplished. We'd practised hard and felt satisfied that we had done our best. It had been a great experience, and we could always try again.

# Going for round two!

In 2013, we decided to audition for series 7 of *Australia's Got Talent*. A lot had changed since our first attempt. We'd just finished high school and were more familiar with the show. We'd become fans of *AGT*, and loved watching the different acts from around Australia compete. So, when we saw that they were holding auditions in Perth, something about the timing felt right. It had been five years since our first appearance, and we knew we'd improved. We were older, more mature and had grown as performers. We were ready.

This time, we entered as ourselves rather than using a stage name. By this point, people at dance competitions had started referring to us as 'the Rybka Twins', so it seemed natural to use our name.

Once again, we had to pre-audition in front of the producers before we could do the TV auditions, and the pre-auditions turned out to be exhausting. We got there early, along with the other acts, but the producers couldn't tell any of us when our turn was going to be, which meant the two of us kept warming up all day. And because we don't like to eat much before we perform, we didn't eat that much. So, we were hungry and warming up until the moment we auditioned, and of course we were, legit, the last performers.

But when we finally got in the room, we were ready. We'd prepared a routine to a Michael Jackson song, and the very first thing the producer said to us was, 'You're not going to be able to use that track on TV because of royalties,'

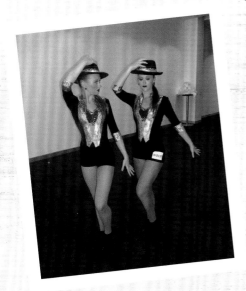

Rehearsing our routine
for probably the 100th
time before our audition
for the producers.

135

but they let us audition with it anyway. It went really well. The producers liked what they saw and said that we had a good chance of getting in. We'd find out in a few weeks whether we'd made it through to the TV round of the auditions.

Eventually, someone from the show rang and said, 'Yep, you're coming back to Perth in a few weeks to film, and you can audition for the judges in front of a live audience.' This was hugely exciting, but the producers wanted us to put together a new routine before then. Not gonna lie, having to create a routine from scratch with only a few weeks before those live TV auditions was scary.

*Every spare second* was spent
rehearsing that *routine.*

• • •

But rather than worry about what we couldn't control, we focused on finding the perfect song. We wanted to create a routine that everyone would enjoy and be able to relate to—we listened to so many songs in the car trying to find the right one! We kept coming back to a few, and eventually, Mum suggested 'Pound the Alarm' by Nicki Minaj. After playing it over and over, we all agreed it was the one. Mum did the choreography and then we put it all together and practised and practised and practised. Every spare second was spent rehearsing that routine.

The live TV auditions were held at the Perth Convention and Exhibition Centre. We got there early in the morning and signed in. Right when we arrived, the TV team miked us up, and told us we'd have to keep these little microphones on all day (even in the toilets, eek!). All of this was new to us. They sat us down to film a little mini-interview, and we were both so camera-shy; we hated it. Neither of us really knew what to say. (It's funny to think that we talk to a camera almost every day now!)

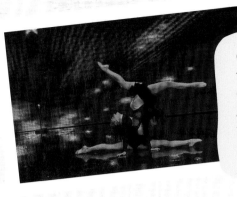

Go to YouTube to view our 'Australia's Got Talent 2013 | Auditions | The Rybka Twins Bend Their Bodies' video.

*This experience changed our lives.*

We knew quite a few of the acts auditioning that day. It was so nice to have people we knew around and to perform on home ground. Lots of our friends and family came out to support us in the audience—some even made signs and held them up (you can see them if you watch the clips on YouTube!).

When it was finally our turn to perform, the routine went really well. The music started, and everything just clicked and came together. It was over before we knew it. The audience clapped and cheered the whole way through our performance and even gave us a standing ovation at the end. Standing on stage afterwards, we both felt so proud of how everything had gone. We were on such a high because we felt so much love for what we were doing . . . it was the most incredible feeling.

The judges gave us good feedback, too, which we hadn't necessarily expected. That year, there were four judges: Timomatic, Kyle Sandilands, Dawn French and Geri Halliwell. An acro troupe we knew had auditioned before us and mentioned that Geri hadn't liked them because she 'hated acro'. So, before we even went on stage, we were bracing ourselves for a negative comment from her. But during our performance, she started nodding her head and getting into it a bit. Her comment to us was something like, 'You're actually pretty good.' We were like, 'Oh my gosh, we won her over!' We couldn't have hoped for better responses from the other judges; Dawn, Kyle and Timomatic had such nice things to say about the routine. We were on top of the world with four yesses!

But, in a repeat of our first time on the show, the producers explained that they were going to need to cull a few acts, so we'd have to go home and wait for that phone call. Since everything had gone so well, we felt we had a good chance of making it through this time. But, a couple of weeks later, Mum got a phone call while we were at uni. She had to break it to us that we hadn't made it through after all that hard work and hoping. (Pretty sure we cried!)

One of the lessons we learned here is that life is unpredictable, because a week or two after that 'no' call, Mum got another phone call from one of the producers who'd seen us do our original Michael Jackson routine. He said something along the lines of, 'We want to give you a chance on the show.' Obviously, we were over the moon. Talk about a roller-coaster! It was probably an even better feeling than being told 'yes' straight away!

A note from ... *Sam*

I remember being on the train and getting a call from Mum where she just said, 'I've got some news for you.' I had no idea what it could be, but it didn't even cross my mind for a second that it would be about the show. And then, when we both got in the car with her at the train station, she told us that we were going to be on the next round of *AGT,* and we both started screaming and yelling. We just couldn't believe it. We were so excited!

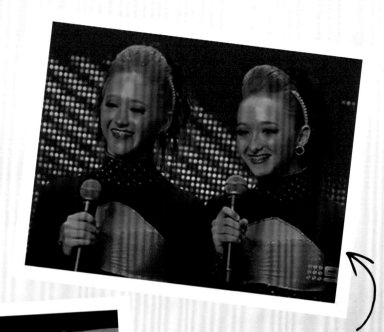

Talking to the judges after performing.

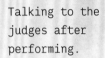

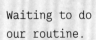

Waiting to do our routine.

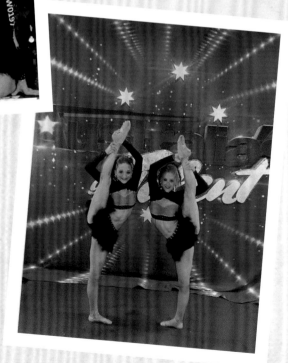

The next round was being filmed in Sydney, so we got to fly there, and that was exciting in itself. But because we were a late addition to this round, we only had a few weeks to come up with a totally new routine! Again, we struggled to find a song. We'd find one we liked, send it to the producers, and they'd come back to say no, they couldn't clear it for use on TV. To add to the pressure, they told us they were going to need us to perform earlier than expected! Our prep time had shrunk from five or six weeks to two weeks. (Seriously, the most stressful two weeks of our lives!) Thankfully, they let us know that any Lady Gaga song would be fine, so we were happy about that because we're big fans and had even seen her in concert. We ended up going with a medley of 'Judas' and 'Americano'.

The thing we remember most about those weeks is how tired we were. We were at uni, so we were going to our classes, coming home and practising every spare moment. But in a way, our lives have always been like that. We just find a way to fit it all in and we never say we can't do something if there's the slightest possibility we can.

Once the music and routine were sorted, we had to create and design our costumes—these ones were really fierce. The dressmaker we go to is pretty quick, and we have a good relationship with her. Usually, what happens is that we get inspiration, mostly from looking online, and then we sketch out designs and take them to her. She'll suggest a few ideas and add her own little touches—she's seriously awesome at giving them that extra sparkle. She often cuts things close, and this time, because the whole thing was super-rushed, things came right down to the very last minute. After staying up all night to finish them, she pulled up outside our house with the costumes minutes before we had to leave for the airport. Now, that's cutting it fine!

*Thanks, Dee! You're the best.*

# Rehearsal blues

We flew into Sydney a few days before filming the semifinal show. One of the first things we had to do once we got to the set was film our on-camera interview. (This still felt so awkward! We weren't used to talking in front of a camera.) The next day was blocked off for practising and fine-tuning everything, and the third day was the actual performance. Each act was given time to practise on the real stage before the semifinal, so we could all get used to the set.

When our allotted rehearsal time came around, things didn't go well. For one thing, getting used to the stage was a big adjustment. Until then, we'd only practised the routine on grass at the oval near our house. Now we needed to get used to doing the tricks on a floor. Usually, when we perform on floors, it's at competitions or for shows where the floors are designed for that purpose—they have a little more give or are sometimes even sprung. This floor was slippery and had no bounce.

The props team had also made us a table prop—at our request— so we could do an aerial off it. We'd been using a brick wall at the oval as a stand-in for the table, but when we rehearsed with the real thing, it was a totally different height to the wall, so we had to adjust to that difference, too.

There was another thing worrying us about that stage—we couldn't grip on it! The huge spotlights over the stage meant there was a lot of dust falling onto it. We felt that the floors needed to be swept before we performed, because the dust on the bottoms of our shoes made everything slippery—the last thing you want when you're performing tricks.

One of the moves in our routine involved putting our hats down in front of us and then using our feet to pick them up. This had gone well whenever we'd practised on grass, but in rehearsal, Sam's hat kept slipping forwards on the stage floor. When things like this start happening the day before a big performance, it's easy to start feeling overwhelmed. We felt so dead. We'd been pushing our bodies so hard practising for this performance that we barely had the energy to get off the floor now that we were there. We also didn't feel safe doing our tricks on the stage floor, so we were racking our brains trying to think of something to help us grip better. Suddenly, Mum came up with this great idea to use Coca-Cola on the soles of our shoes to make them sticky. It actually worked! The wardrobe department ended up having a special sticky tape that we were able to use on the hats to prevent them from sliding on the floor, too, so that was a huge relief. We practised that hat trick over and over until we were sure it would work.

For some reason, the producers rushed us through our rehearsal time, meaning we didn't get the time we'd been promised. After that bad rehearsal, we went back to our hotel feeling pretty disappointed. First we'd gone from four or five weeks of rehearsal time to only two weeks, and now our rehearsal time on stage had been cut, too.

Once we got back to the hotel, Mum rang the producers. 'That went really badly,' she said. 'Can we please come back and get the rehearsal time we were promised?' They agreed, so straight away we turned around and went back to the studio. It was the last thing we wanted to do—we felt so dead—but, at the same time, it was the only thing we wanted to do. We needed to redeem ourselves before the big performance.

At this point in the competition, each act could ask the show's creative team for enhancements, such as lighting or pyrotechnics, to make their actual performance a little more impressive than in the audition round. We didn't know too much about that sort of thing—just what we'd seen from watching previous seasons of the show—but we definitely wanted an explosion and flames at the end of our routine. When we asked for these things, we were told, 'Oh no. You guys don't need anything like that!' And not being experts in this area, we let them talk us out of it.

Thankfully, after that second rehearsal we felt much better about everything. We arrived back at the hotel room, exhausted. That night, Mum and our aunties Linda and Leonie spent hours madly glittering our costumes and setting them with our hair dryers! Mum hadn't been 100 per cent happy with them when she'd seen us wearing them on stage. Luckily, our aunties and our best friend Danielle had all flown in from Perth to watch us the next day, so they were happy to help add those last little touches, which finished off the costumes perfectly.

We went to bed early so we could get a good night's sleep and be well rested for the next day. (Yeah, right!) But obviously, we were so nervous that we just lay awake, worrying. We couldn't help it—we were older and wiser now. We knew if we made a mistake, we weren't going to be able to get away from it. It would be on TV, on YouTube . . . basically everywhere. Everyone we knew was going to be watching. Most of all, we didn't want to let each other down. When we look back now, we think, how did we get through those nerves? But as terrified as we were, we were also excited to showcase our passion and what we love to do. And those feelings almost overtook our nerves. Almost.

## Showtime!

The day of the show, we kept ourselves from getting too scared by refusing to let negative thoughts into our minds. When one of us started getting a little too worried, the other one would start talking about how we could do this, about how much we had practised and practised, and that WE WERE READY.

We were also trying to decide on the perfect time to put the Coke on our shoes, so they'd be the right level of stickiness; we didn't want to put it on too late or too early. We were walking around backstage without our shoes on because Mum had our shoes so she could do the honours. Eventually, it came time to get in position, so we put our sticky shoes on, and the producers took Mum out to the audience. We wanted her to watch us from there so she could tell us later how everything had looked. Suddenly, it was just the two of us waiting to go on. (Argh! We're getting nervous even writing about this now!) We kept telling each other, 'We can do this.' And we stayed positive. You can't ever let yourself get into a negative state of mind, because once you're there, it's hard to get back out.

We got into position, and the lights went down. The huge screen behind the stage began running our interview for the live audience and the judges. We hadn't seen the footage either, so we listened to our interviews as we balanced up on the props—looking at the screens, and then looking at each other . . . and then at that massive audience watching us. It was down to the last 30 seconds before our performance, and it was the craziest thing . . . watching that footage, which included clips of us dancing, got us that little bit more excited. It reminded us of all the work we'd put in to get here. It reminded us of why we were there.

## The performance

Suddenly, the video on the screen ended, the lights went down and the theatre went silent. Those long seconds right before you begin a performance are the longest and scariest because you know the moment has come. There's no turning back. Your heart beats so fast, and the adrenaline kicks in. When you're a performer, there's a fine line between using that energy and letting it conquer you; adrenaline can either help you nail your routine and jump higher, or it can overwhelm you and make you completely fall to pieces. Your job is to walk that line.

When you're dancing, it's important to stay in the moment; it's like being in a semiconscious state. If you're thinking about what you have to do and are in your head too much, then you aren't 'doing' it. This is when things can go wrong. By the time you get on stage, you should have practised so much that you're able to enjoy yourself and let go. Dancing means so much to us because when we're dancing it's just music, movement and us . . . nothing else matters.

We've always said to each other that whatever happens during a performance, we mustn't let each other down. If something goes wrong, just let it go and make the next step even better. Don't dwell on the mistake, and don't let the people watching remember that you made a mistake. But luckily, nothing went wrong in this performance, which we are so grateful for! Before we knew it, the moment was over, the audience was cheering, and it was done.

Each of the judges said our performance was pretty much perfect. The one negative comment was from Kyle, who said that it had missed a big finish. And he was right! Even the lighting had gone softer near the end of our performance, and without an explosion or other big moment, it had felt like a big build-up for nothing. We stood there and smiled as we listened, but inside we were thinking, 'We did ask for that!' But it was too late by then.

Dawn said that we'd managed to win her over again, which was really nice. And Timomatic said we were world-class, the best in the competition and deserved a spot in the grand final!

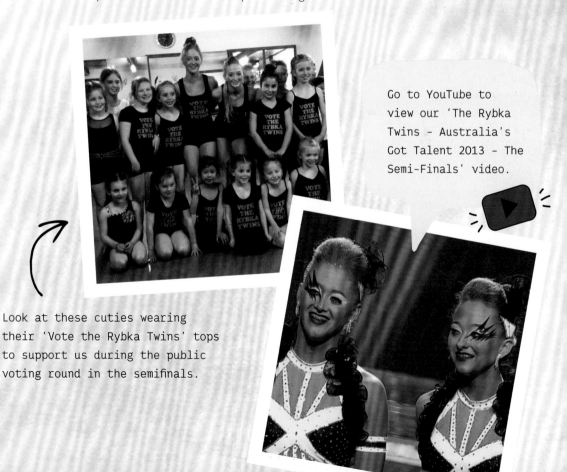

Go to YouTube to view our 'The Rybka Twins - Australia's Got Talent 2013 - The Semi-Finals' video.

Look at these cuties wearing their 'Vote the Rybka Twins' tops to support us during the public voting round in the semifinals.

# The final performances

Because we made it to the top three in that semifinal group, we were flown back to appear at the beginning of the next round. This stage of the competition was based on viewer votes. The act with the highest number of votes made it straight through to the next round, and the judges would decide who went through out of the two acts left. We were happy to make it to that stage, but unfortunately we didn't make it through. It was between us and a hip-hop crew, and they chose the crew.

After we filmed that round, it was over. We were back in a taxi and then on a plane back to Perth. It was a pretty sad plane ride home. But a couple of weeks later, we were asked to fly back to perform in the grand final with some of the other acts who'd appeared on the show. We flew back to Sydney for the third time that month. This time,

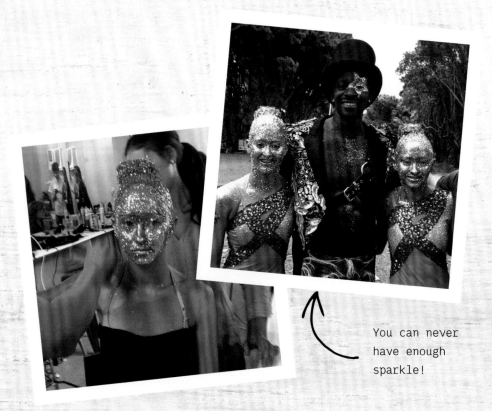

You can never have enough sparkle!

the pressure was off, and we just wanted to have fun and do our best. We were given a slot of the music that would be used in the group performance to choreograph something for, and then once we got to Sydney, a choreographer worked with all the acts to tell us when to come in, and what to do with the other performers.

As part of our mini-routine, we got to perform contortion tricks on stands that lifted up to the roof of the theatre; it was fun! But at the end, when the pyrotechnics went off below us, we couldn't breathe because of all the smoke! When we came down, we looked at each other and said, 'Did you think you were going to die just now?' . . . 'I did!'

We had to do our own hair for the performances, but the hair and make-up team helped us out with makeup for the cameras. After they'd finished with us, Mum thought we needed glitter in our hair, because we always had that extra sparkle in our hair for comps. She put glitter in our hair and the hair, and make-up guy was so angry! He was mad at Mum for adding to what he'd done.

## We just wanted to *have fun* and do our best.

• • •

We don't know if it was revenge for Mum's 'glittervention' or not, but the following week, when the show's team did our hair and make-up, they covered our entire necks and faces with glitter and paint. We didn't quite know what to say, so there we were, walking around backstage with all this glitter all over our faces and hair. Everyone who passed us did a double take and said, 'What the heck?' when they saw us. Even Timomatic came out of his dressing room and said, 'What is going on?' when he saw our faces. During the dress rehearsal, while we were sitting in the audience and Julia Morris was on stage practising her lines, she kept making comments about our faces because we looked so ridiculous. LOL!

## A learning experience

Although we hadn't achieved the result we wanted, being on
the show taught us a lot. We both improved so much, especially
throughout the 2013 series, because we practised every single day.
Getting all those tricks right meant we were able to do them perfectly,
whenever we wanted. They almost became automatic.

We also learned how much effort and rehearsal time it takes
to prepare for a performance at that level. The difference between
our levels of strength and flexibility in the beginning of the audition
process and at the final performance was huge. Having those
big performances to work towards helped us to push ourselves
that much further.

## The *AGT* effect

Appearing on *Australia's Got Talent* in 2013 was a turning point for
us. A lot of dancers and acrobats saw us on that show. At the time we
filmed it, neither of us had Instagram or Twitter (which surprises a lot
of people!), but the show's producers wanted us to start accounts so
we'd be able to help promote the shows when they aired.

That's why we got on Instagram, which was the beginning of
everything we have today. People started following us and, suddenly,
it felt as though more and more people knew who we were.

One day we went to a workshop with a teacher from Melbourne,
and she said, 'Everyone in Melbourne is talking about you.' We couldn't
believe it—we were oblivious to anything outside the dance world in
Perth. Then, in 2014, Abby Lee Miller from the TV show *Dance Moms*
came to Australia to hold dance masterclasses. We are huge fans of
*Dance Moms* (more on that in chapter 7), so we flew to Melbourne to
go to a class. It was there that we noticed people recognising us from
*Australia's Got Talent*. Girls stopped us and asked for photos—some
even approached us in the bathroom! It was overwhelming in a way,
but we also loved it. And that was only the beginning.

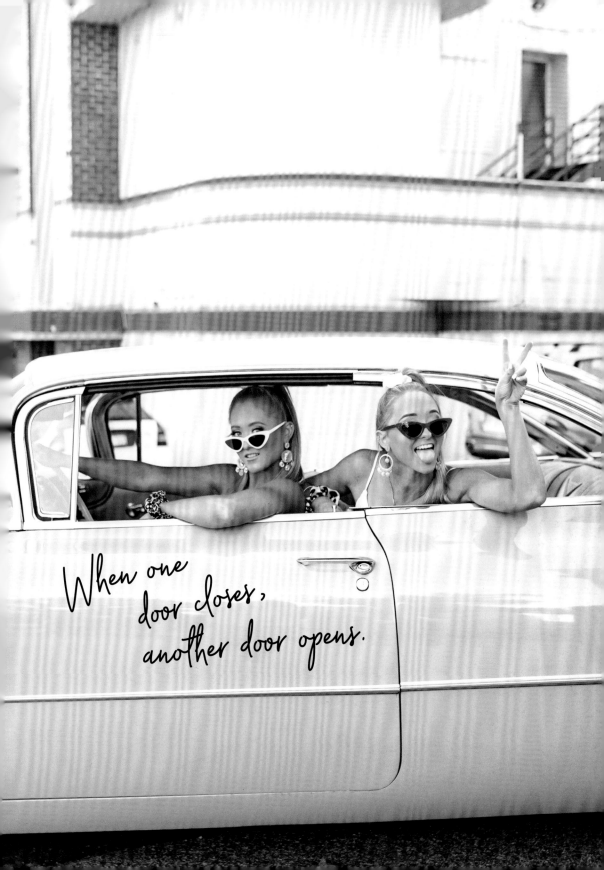

When one
door closes,
another door opens.

# CHAPTER 7

# Dance Moms

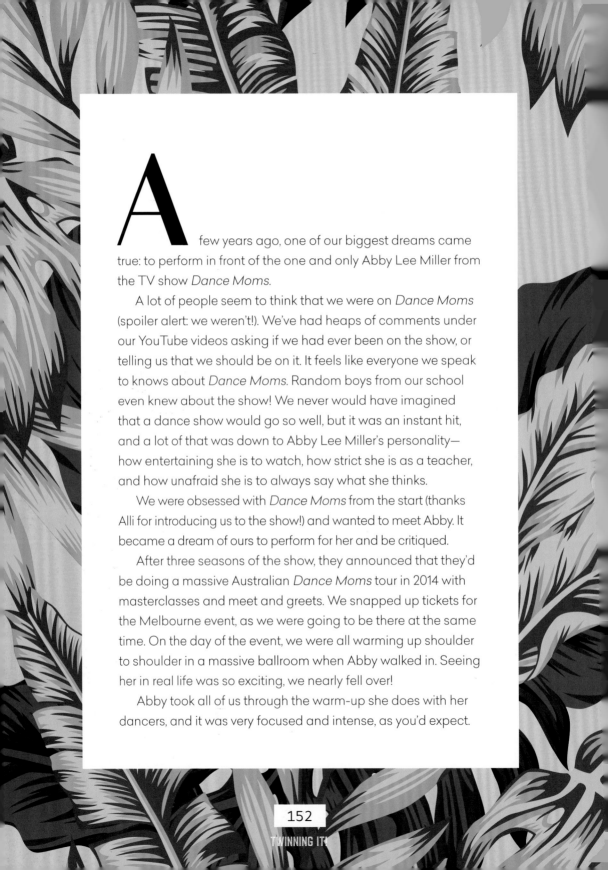

A few years ago, one of our biggest dreams came true: to perform in front of the one and only Abby Lee Miller from the TV show *Dance Moms*.

A lot of people seem to think that we were on *Dance Moms* (spoiler alert: we weren't!). We've had heaps of comments under our YouTube videos asking if we had ever been on the show, or telling us that we should be on it. It feels like everyone we speak to knows about *Dance Moms*. Random boys from our school even knew about the show! We never would have imagined that a dance show would go so well, but it was an instant hit, and a lot of that was down to Abby Lee Miller's personality— how entertaining she is to watch, how strict she is as a teacher, and how unafraid she is to always say what she thinks.

We were obsessed with *Dance Moms* from the start (thanks Alli for introducing us to the show!) and wanted to meet Abby. It became a dream of ours to perform for her and be critiqued.

After three seasons of the show, they announced that they'd be doing a massive Australian *Dance Moms* tour in 2014 with masterclasses and meet and greets. We snapped up tickets for the Melbourne event, as we were going to be there at the same time. On the day of the event, we were all warming up shoulder to shoulder in a massive ballroom when Abby walked in. Seeing her in real life was so exciting, we nearly fell over!

Abby took all of us through the warm-up she does with her dancers, and it was very focused and intense, as you'd expect.

The first of
many photos
with the one
and only Abby
Lee Miller.

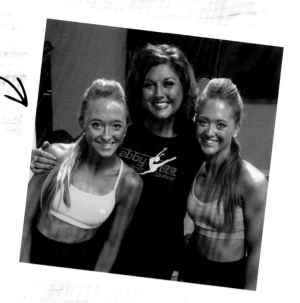

A quick snap on stage
after the Adelaide
masterclass.

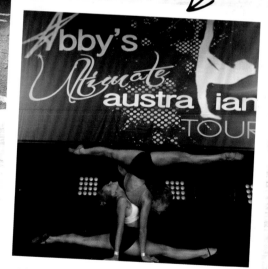

With Kendall Vertes and
Maddie Ziegler outside
the dance studio in LA
where they were filming
*Dance Moms*.

After that, Gianna taught us some choreography, and at the end of the session we performed the choreography in groups in front of Abby. We were told we could improvise our own moves for this bit, so of course we whipped out our acro tricks. We were so excited when Abby chose both of us to go through to the next round.

For that round, each of us had to sing in front of everyone, which was totally unexpected. There were so many people in the ballroom. Abby handed Sam the microphone first, and Sam just did it! She started singing, and she sounded pretty good. But when it was Teagan's turn, she totally froze!

A note from ... *Teagan*

I did! I couldn't think of anything to sing! I was still trying to get over the shock of seeing Sam sing in front of all those people. When Abby passed me the microphone, I started singing 'Happy Birthday'. (Oh no!) It was the worst, but at least I tried and didn't say I wouldn't do it, or that I couldn't think of a song. A few people did that, and they got knocked out automatically. Even if you sounded awful, you had to be willing to have a go. That's an awesome lesson everyone can learn.

Teagan got knocked out, but Sam made it through to the next round, where Abby asked her to do a side aerial—which she smashed. Next, Abby asked all the girls say their age. When Sam said 'seventeen', Abby knocked her out because it was too old. She said to Sam that if she was ever asked that question again she should ask, 'What age do you want me to be?'

After this, they had a meet and greet with photos. By the time our turn came around, the crowds had disappeared and our friend Ashi Ross, and her teacher Rebecca Davies, who'd come to the event with us, asked us to come backstage. Ashi had met the *Dance Moms* cast before, so we were lucky to have that connection. When we got backstage, they were all there: Abby, the girls and their mothers—the actual dance moms! It was pretty much the coolest experience we'd ever had.

We were on such a *high* from meeting all the *people* we'd loved watching on TV *for years!*

• • •

Abby was nice and asked us so many questions. She wanted to know who our coach was, and was really interested when we told her it was our mum. Abby wanted to meet her, so we got Mum and brought her backstage, too. She wanted to see our performance from *Australia's Got Talent,* so we showed it to her. Meeting Abby was the cherry on top of an amazing day. We walked all the way home to the hotel instead of taking a taxi because we were on such a high from meeting all the people we'd loved watching on TV for years!

In 2015, the tour came back, and this time we ended up flying to the masterclass in Adelaide. We were lined up outside the auditorium when the girls from the show drove by and waved at everyone. Suddenly, Maddie spotted us and quickly ran up to give us a hug. She was so friendly and down-to-earth. We were so happy that she'd remembered us! Once we got inside, Abby also spotted us and was excited to see us; it was so nice—like seeing old friends.

At this event, if you made it to the top ten of the group, you got to perform a solo in front of Abby and some of the girls. This was a big opportunity. We started with Abby's warm-up and then all of us learned a combo, which we'd be able to improvise on in the end dance. The next round was ballet, and the ballet combo Abby taught us was tough. We love ballet, but because Abby is big on technique, she didn't demonstrate the steps, she just used the correct terms for them. Thankfully, we made it through to the next round, where each of us had to improvise a dance to whatever genre Abby called out, with no music.

A note from ... *Sam*

Teagan wasn't about to make the same mistake again, so this time, she was fully prepared to sing if she needed to. On the plane, she'd practised the same song over and over. And it was lucky she was ready, because Abby asked all of the finalists to sing again.

Finally, it was the moment we'd been dreaming of: we each got to perform a one-minute solo in front of Abby and some of the *Dance Moms* dancers. Teagan's solo went down really well. Abby even told her, 'You've carved out a niche for yourself.' Sam's solo also went super well and got positive comments. Abby said she kept her on the edge of her seat throughout the performance, and she loved the choreography.

The girls were so good at critiquing us. Abby had obviously taught them well. After watching Abby on TV week after week, we had both been desperate to know what she'd say after seeing us perform. Even now, we can't quite believe we got that opportunity. Abby's comments were very positive, which was cool because with

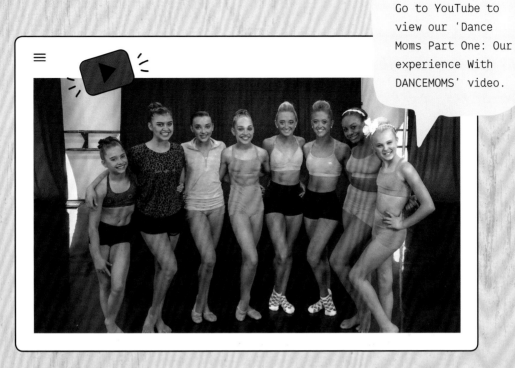

Go to YouTube to view our 'Dance Moms Part One: Our experience With DANCEMOMS' video.

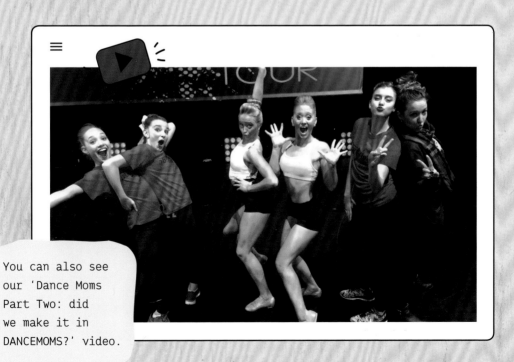

You can also see our 'Dance Moms Part Two: did we make it in DANCEMOMS?' video.

Abby, you just never know—she could have critiqued us a lot. That's the risk you take by putting yourself out there.

After the solos, Abby announced this was going to be part of a national competition, and that she'd be choosing some of us to go to Melbourne the following weekend to compete in her Ultimate Dance Competition. She also told us it would be filmed and aired as part of the *Dance Moms* show. And we were chosen! We couldn't believe we were actually going to be on an episode of our favourite show.

The next weekend, we flew to Melbourne, and we were so nervous. Even though this was our third experience of filming for a TV show, it was just as nerve-racking. When we were all assembled, Abby explained what would be happening: we would each have an interview with her (her advice was to not use the word 'um'). After the interviews, we'd do our solo performances, and then she'd announce the winners. She said, 'You've got one shot. Make it count.'

## The whole experience ranks as one of the *craziest* and most *exciting* things we've been a part of.

• • •

On the night of the performance, there were cameras everywhere and Abby was sitting right in front of the stage. Sam performed a jazz solo and Teagan did an acro solo. Both of us felt happy with our performances, and at the end of the comp, Teagan was named Abby's Ultimate Senior Dancer. This blew our minds; it was a really big achievement.

In the end, it turned out that the episodes filmed in Australia wouldn't be aired on TV after all. (Gutted!) It felt like a carrot had been dangled in front of us and snatched away. But even so, the experience ranks as one of the most exciting things we've been a part of.

Since then, we've stayed in touch with Abby through social media and have met up at different times. When we've been in LA, she's invited us to the set of *Dance Moms* and even asked us to teach an acro workshop at her studio, which was so fun. Another time, when we were in the United States after winning a scholarship for the Joffrey Ballet School, we were at a movie premiere—we'd been invited by our friend Haley Huelsman, who danced with Abby and then with Candy Apple's—and Abby spotted us. When she stood up to make a speech, she started talking about us and then asked us to pop up on stage and do an acro trick for the audience (which, of course, we did). Bottom line: when it comes to Abby, always be ready for the unexpected! It's been really special getting to know her—she's so interesting to listen to, and has so many amazing stories.

Whenever we think back to our favourite memories, or things we've accomplished, we always go to *Australia's Got Talent* and all of our experiences with the cast of *Dance Moms*. These are things we are so grateful for, and moments we'll remember forever.

These experiences also reflect what we've learned about show business in general: big opportunities can come up out of nowhere, but sometimes things you are promised won't end up happening. Things change quickly in entertainment. You've got to be prepared to do things that make you nervous, but also be prepared for them not to happen. You take the ups with the downs. If something that's been promised happens, great! If it doesn't, shrug it off and keep going until the next opportunity comes along.

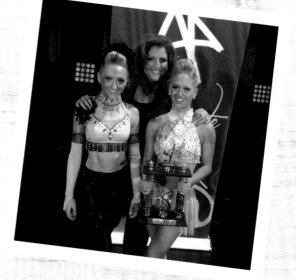

A very special moment after Teagan was named Ultimate Senior Dancer.

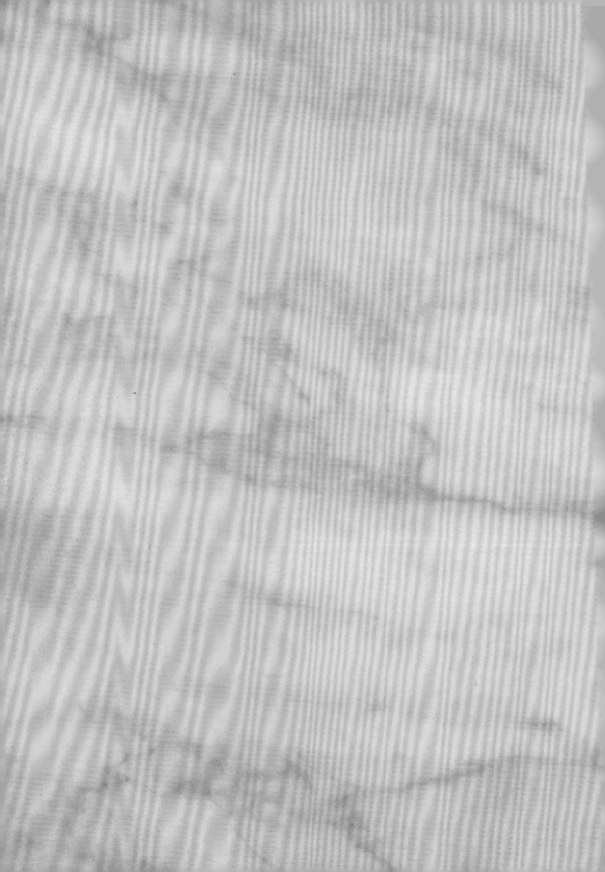

# CHAPTER 8

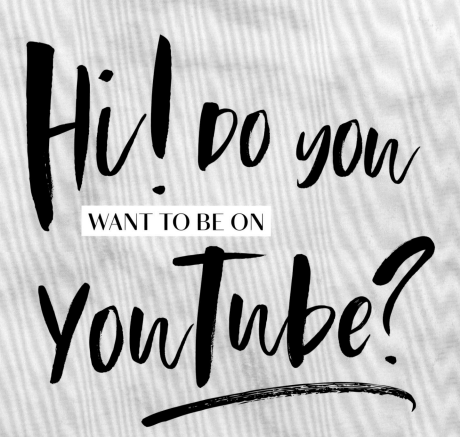

Hi! Do you
WANT TO BE ON
YouTube?

Creating content for our social media accounts and interacting with our amazing followers and subscribers is a way of life for us now; it's something we love doing. Posting videos and pics has become second nature to us, and more unbelievably, it's even become our full-time careers!

Because of this, people are often surprised when they find out that we were actually late to the whole social media thing (like, really late!). We were the last ones in our friend group to get Instagram, and the only reason we even started those accounts was because the producers from *Australia's Got Talent* encouraged us to after we appeared on the show, so we could promote the episodes when they aired. We never imagined having so many followers, or that this would be something we could do for a living. It all happened by accident.

After our second go on *Australia's Got Talent,* we started getting a bit more recognised, which was fun and new, but we didn't think that much of it. It felt like a novelty that would pass, and we were just going along for the ride. We still had three years of university ahead of us, so we were totally focused on our degrees and our dancing.

But once we started using Instagram in particular, we were both like, 'Oh, this is pretty cool!' It's one of our favourite apps now, and we get so much inspiration from it. We have to be careful though, because time disappears whenever we're on it. #timesucker! (Don't go on Instagram if you've got stuff to do!)

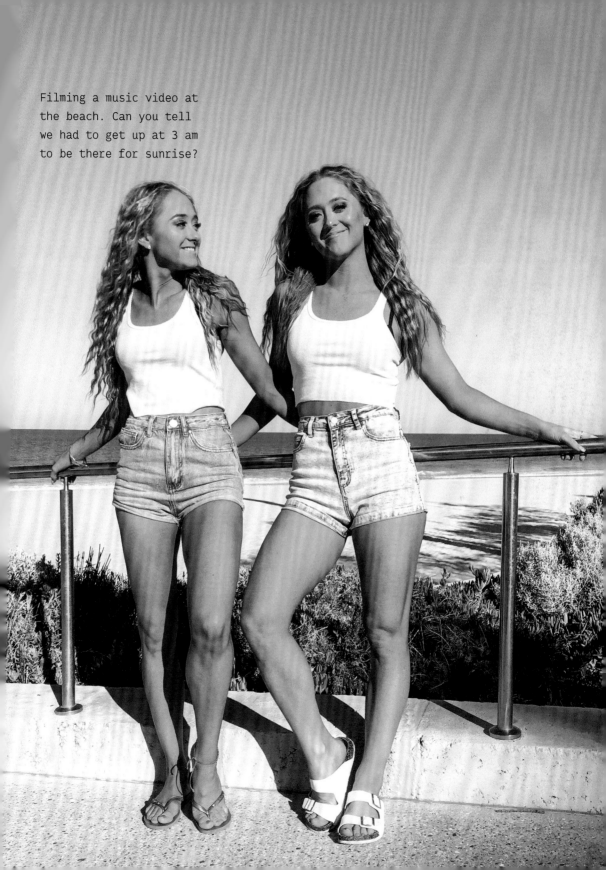

Filming a music video at the beach. Can you tell we had to get up at 3 am to be there for sunrise?

Bit by bit, people began to find us on Instagram. And then, after *Australia's Got Talent* aired, we noticed an influx of new followers on our accounts. This motivated us to keep posting—now that people were following us, we thought we'd better give them something to follow! Whenever we went somewhere interesting, we'd do acro poses and post them. And we'd go all-out on special holidays by dressing up in the theme of that day, then posting pics of us doing acro in costume. Lots of people seemed to like these types of posts and our accounts continued to grow as more people kept finding us.

Back then, we were probably posting once a week, but now we pretty much post every night. The more followers and likes we got, the more encouraged we were to keep going and think of new ideas. We think it's so cool whenever someone decides to follow us—and people who comment on our posts tell us so many interesting things. We love it when people feel inspired by the things we do, or tell us that we're the reason they tried dance or acro. We also get messages saying things like, 'I was feeling really down today, but then you guys posted your video and after I watched it, I felt so happy. Thanks for putting that up.' Messages like those motivate us to keep going. All we're doing is sharing something we love with the world, so to find out that we're helping people in some way, making them smile or inspiring them to try new things, makes it so much more satisfying.

# The internet ... a weird and wonderful place!

Before we tell you how we got started on Instagram and YouTube, we want to talk about internet safety because it's such a big concern these days. There are so many great things you can do online, but it's also true that certain areas of the internet come with their own dangers, and it's smart to be aware of them.

If you're under eighteen years old and posting online, keeping your profile private is one of the best ways to keep yourself safe: that way, you know exactly who is following you, and you can control who looks at your account. Always check with a parent before posting any content; they love you and are there to look out for you, so they're the best judge of what's safe and appropriate for you to put online.

We didn't grow up with social media, so having to talk to our parents about what we were doing online was never an issue for us. We were in Year 10 when we got Facebook, which was a big thing back then. By the time we started posting on Instagram and YouTube, we were older. If we'd been younger, Mum would have been very strict about what we could be on and what we could post. And we would have been okay with her being involved, because it's important for parents to be aware of that stuff.

We've always had an open relationship with our mum, and we know that she's just trying to protect us. Everyone should feel they have someone older and more experienced in life to turn to. The things you say and post on social media shouldn't be anything that you need to keep private from your parents. If your mum or dad wants to see your phone so they know what you've been doing online, you shouldn't feel that you can't show them. You shouldn't be doing anything that you don't want them to see anyway—at least that's how we feel about it. We have nothing to hide.

Even if you're an older teenager with a smartphone and all the answers in the world at your fingertips, that doesn't mean you necessarily know how to respond when someone messages you inappropriately. You might think something is fine to post, but then realise later it wasn't a good idea. It's natural not to think about serious consequences when you're young; that's why it's important to have an adult's input.

If someone posts a mean comment about you or messages you something that doesn't feel right, tell your parents right away. We find the best thing to do is to then block that person so you don't know or see anything they're doing, and they can't see your posts. People who write negative comments just want your attention and are trying to get a reaction. Ignore them and block them, and you'll find that they just move on when they don't get what they want. The internet shouldn't be a negative place, but on some level, you always have to be aware of risks when you're online. It's not a perfect world.

## Stay private, guys!

Even if you're over eighteen, have a public account and can post whatever you like, it's still safer to keep some things to yourself. When the two of us are out and we post things on Instagram, we very rarely post the location of where we are. The only thing we might tag is the state we are in, or the city—but we won't tag the specific café or the beach because we think that's a pretty personal thing. You don't want people you haven't met knowing where you go to school or where you hang out.

Our last tip is to always be careful if you're messaging someone you haven't met. You might think you're messaging a thirteen-year-old, but who knows who's really behind the keyboard? It could be someone with less straightforward intentions. (Scary thought, but it happens all the time.)

Bottom line: keep yourself safe online. Be smart about your posts, and you'll be able to enjoy all the fun things about being online, which is how it should be!

## Opportunities can come out of nowhere

Around the same time we started our Insta account, we also got a Twitter account (again, because the TV producers encouraged us to get one), but we never got that into Twitter. Even now, we pretty much never use it. To be honest, we find it confusing (LOL!). Katy Perry loves it though (and we love her!), so occasionally we go on there. But it did bring us a major opportunity.

# *Block* **THE BULLIES**

A big chunk of everyone's lives is spent on the internet now and, because of that, bullying is a problem on social media accounts and DMs. Some of the cyber-bullying stories we hear are so awful; we just can't believe people can be like that. It makes us want to stand up and say that this is a no-bullying zone.

We recently experienced online hate when someone accused us of doing something that we didn't do. She tagged us on her social media, and suddenly, we were getting all these horrible comments and we didn't know why. Eventually, we found out and went straight to this person to clear up the misunderstanding. We took down our post because we wanted to be sensitive to her concerns, but it didn't really resolve the situation. Many people writing the nasty comments didn't know the full story—they were just keyboard warriors, saying things they'd probably never say to our faces. Regardless, it's hard not to take those things personally. If someone starts sending you mean comments and you're under eighteen, tell an adult right away. Then block the commenter(s) from your account, so they can't see or say anything about your life.

Growing up, Mum always told us to treat people the way we wanted to be treated. Another one of her favourite sayings was, 'If you haven't got anything nice to say, don't say anything at all.' She was exactly right. There's no need for any of that meanness or negativity.

In 2015, we got a message on Twitter from twins in the United States named Brooklyn and Bailey. They have their own YouTube channel (BrooklynandBailey) and are crazy popular. We'd heard of them before because their mum also has a YouTube channel where she posts hair tutorials (CuteGirlsHairStyles), and we'd watched her videos. We also knew of Brooklyn and Bailey because people on Instagram often told us we looked like them. So, naturally, we had to check them out! (We don't think we look like them, other than that they're twins, too! But I guess that reminds people of us.)

In their message, Brooklyn and Bailey said they were starting a YouTube channel called Squared with twins from around the world, and asked if we would like to be part of it. To be honest, we thought this message was fake. We were like, 'Nah, these girls are too well known. Someone must be scamming us.' But then we found out it was for real, and they did want us to be on their new channel. They said they found us from our *Australia's Got Talent* videos. Crazy how one thing leads to another!

Becoming YouTubers had never crossed our minds. So, once we realised this was real, our initial reaction was . . . no way! The thought of putting ourselves out there every week seemed too scary. It takes a lot to get in front of a camera and make something that the whole world, including all your friends and family, are going to see.

But once we had a chance to think things through, we realised that this was a cool opportunity, and one we probably shouldn't turn down. We agreed to be on Squared for six months to see how it went. We jumped into the YouTube world with no idea how things worked behind the scenes.

Brooklyn, Bailey and their parents, Mindy and Shaun, were so good to us during this time. They walked us through the whole YouTube process and were very supportive. They'd give us a theme to work with for each video, and then each twin group on Squared would put their own touch on it. Having themes to work with really helped in those early days. It meant we didn't have that added pressure of coming up with content ideas right from the start.

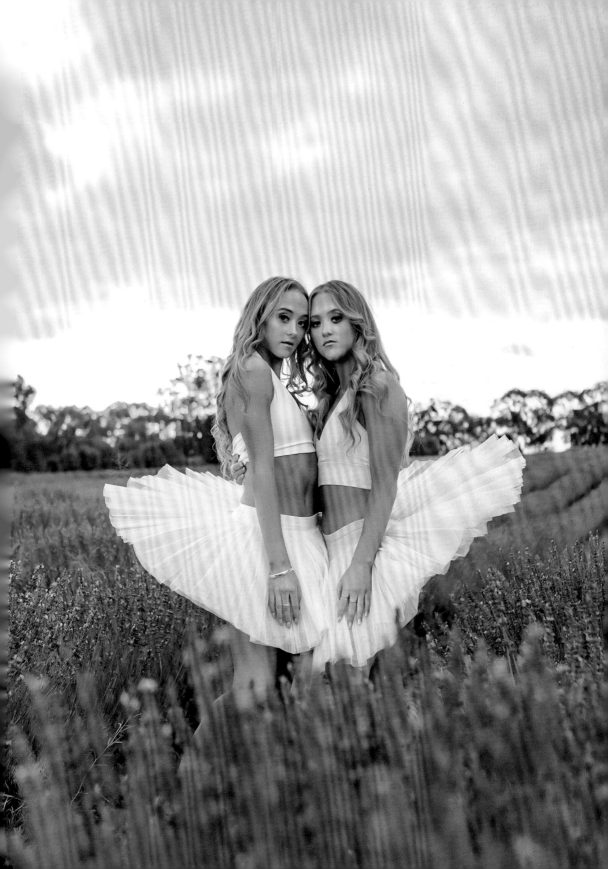

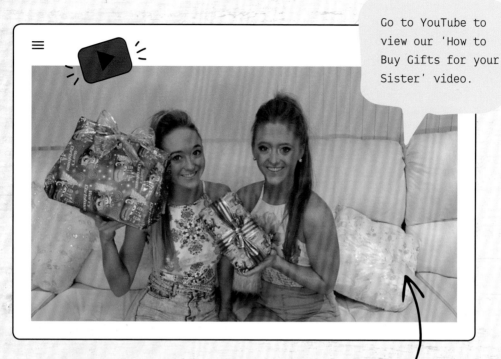

Go to YouTube to view our 'How to Buy Gifts for your Sister' video.

## The first of our 3 am videos!

Because our first video for Squared was due to go up around Christmas, the first theme we were given was 'gifting'. This might sound like an easy theme, but trying to think of a video idea around gifting was actually hard for us! We racked our brains for ages. What does 'gifting' even mean? Finally, we came up with an idea: we'd buy each other a gift and exchange them on camera. The reason we thought this would make a cool video was that we'd never given each other a gift before. (Say whaaaaat?!)

That gifting video was a first for us in lots of ways: it was the first (and only) time we've exchanged gifts, and it was also the first time we'd filmed ourselves talking to the camera. It took us hours to film this video—we're talking all day. Because we weren't used to being in front of a camera, we just kept laughing; neither of us knew what to say and we stuffed up our lines so many times. We probably taped our introduction about fifty million times because we couldn't figure out how we wanted to be, how much energy we should have, what our niche was or what style of video intro suited us. On top of that, we had very little experience with camera equipment, so that slowed us down, too.

The one battery we had for our camera died after a couple of hours of filming, and we had to wait for three hours while it recharged. By the time we finished filming the video, it was 3 am. In fact, most of our first videos for Squared were probably finished around that time; the early videos always seemed to take us all day.

One time, we were given the theme of 'snow day'. Since we don't get snow in Perth, we decided to dress up as Elsa and Anna from *Frozen*, and we were in those costumes all day and night filming that video. Once again, our camera battery kept dying, so we ended up sitting around in those costumes waiting for it to recharge and then we'd go again, then we'd wait for the battery and go again . . . There was also a cooking bit in that video, so we also had to wait for the food to cook. It was a loooong time to be in a *Frozen* costume!

# We don't do gifts!

Some people are shocked when they find out we don't give gifts to each other, but because we're always together and we share so many things, exchanging gifts feels too much like buying presents for ourselves. Maybe later, when we live more separate lives, we'll buy each other gifts. Who knows?

Go to YouTube to view our 'Frozen's Elsa & Anna in Australia' video.

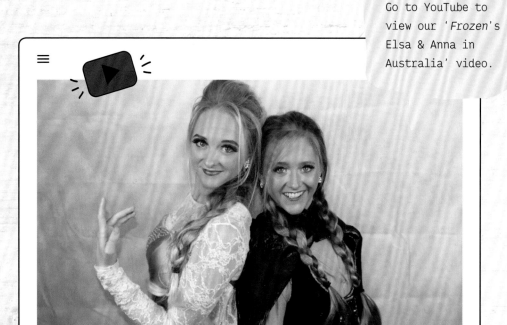

We learned a lot as we went, and, luckily for us, Mindy and Shaun shared so many YouTube tips with us, such as telling us which cameras were good to use, and explaining how to get good lighting. They didn't tell us to go out and spend a lot of money; they just gave us good advice and were always there to help when we had questions (which was often!). They guided us a lot through those first couple of months on YouTube, and we are so thankful to them.

We dragged a *massive light* out of Dad's shed and stuck it on a stack of *milk crates* and *pillows!*

• • •

At this point, we didn't have any fancy lighting—and forget those flashy ring lights YouTubers use to make themselves look good on

172

camera. We just dragged a massive light out of Dad's shed and stuck it on top of a stack of milk crates and pillows! It was a very DIY job. We didn't have a budget at this point, and we wouldn't encourage anyone new to YouTube to invest a lot of money into equipment, at least not at the beginning.

People often ask us what camera we use. We use a Canon video camera, but you can definitely start with a smartphone. It doesn't pick up sounds as well as a vlogging camera if you're in noisy places, but it's a good way to start until you know if you want to keep filming videos or turn it into more than a hobby.

To make sure we were on time for Squared's posting schedule, we had to film two videos in advance each month. We'd have one week to film, and then a week to edit, but we struggled so much with editing the videos because, back then, we had no idea how to use the editing program.

## ROOKIE TUBER TIP

It's kind of funny now that we look back on it, but even though these videos took hours and hours to film, it never occurred to us to buy extra batteries for our camera. Truth is, we never knew you could! We thought you got the one battery that came with the camera and that was it. Now we have three or four batteries, so those hours of waiting for a battery to recharge are over. If you're into videos and think you'll be making a lot of them, this might be something to think about spending your money on.

# Editing is everything!

The editing process still takes us a very long time, but at least now we know what we're doing. We often come home with two hours of footage to edit, plus we'll have to drop in music, sound effects and sometimes pictures . . . it can be a lot! Because our free time is limited, people often ask, 'Why don't you pay someone to edit your videos?' But we don't want that—we'd be giving up too much control. When we're creating a video, we are the ones with the vision. In our minds, we know exactly what vibe we are trying to get across, and what we want the viewers to see. Nobody else could have the same eyes or the same approach we do, so editing our videos ourselves, even though it's time-consuming, just feels better for us.

If something isn't working, we'll all get together—both of us and Mum—and try to fix it. But in the whole time we've been making videos, we've only had to trash a video once. When it came time to edit it, we watched the footage and it just didn't feel true to us, so we thought, 'Nah, let's start again and film another video.' But 99 per cent of the time, we can find a way to edit around a problem to make the video work. That's why editing is so important.

# Busy days

Around the time we started posting videos on Squared, we were also part of a show touring several Australian cities. It was called the Edge of Dreams Tour, and it featured three dance groups: us, a group of amazing dancers called the Dream Team and a duo from the United States—two really nice girls from the Candy Apple's dance troupe, who were on the show *Dance Moms*, and who we'd met before. The whole tour was an amazing experience for us, but because it coincided with the beginning of our YouTube journey, we didn't get too much time to sightsee in the cities we visited.

We were on the Melbourne leg of the tour when it came time to edit our first video for Squared. Everyone else from the tour was having fun

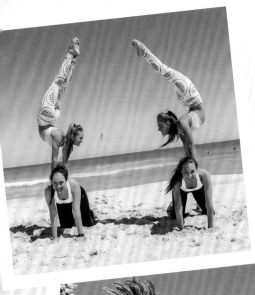

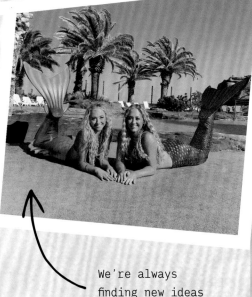

We're always finding new ideas for Instagram and YouTube.

## WE REALISED WE LOVED TOURING

The Edge of Dreams Tour was organised by a company that makes tracksuits and uniforms for dance schools. We'd contacted them because we wanted our own personalised tracksuits, but they asked if we'd be interested in doing this dance tour. It was unexpected, but ended up being so much fun, and it made us realise how much we love performing with other groups as part of a tour.

Being in a different city every few days and performing in front of big audiences was amazing. Plus, we got to experience all of this with other acts who love performing just as much as we do. We made friends with the other girls on tour and had fun ... when we weren't editing videos in our hotel room!

Eventually, we want to go on tour and perform live in front of people again. We can't wait to get out there and say thank you to everyone who's supported us, so we hope it happens soon!

and going out in the city, and there we were, sitting in our hotel room looking up editing tutorials on YouTube! But we knew we couldn't miss our deadline, and we also knew we were going to have to figure out this editing process in order to do the rest of the videos. That edit took a very long time, and this was a pretty stressful time. As well as the tour and starting out on YouTube, we also had uni work we had to do, too.

As time-consuming as those first videos were to film and edit, though, it never crossed our minds to give up. We'd committed to Squared for six months, so we were always going to stick that out—it's not in our nature to quit. Like most things in our life, if we're struggling, we just push through until we aren't struggling anymore.

By the end of our six-month contract with Squared, we were that little bit better on camera, that little bit faster at editing and had learned a lot more about filming. And the best thing was that we were really enjoying making the videos. But because we were in our last year of uni, we had our massive full-on prac coming up, which meant we'd be teaching drama and dance at a high school for ten weeks!

We depend on *dance* to get us through *stressful* times.

• • •

Our uni teachers strongly encouraged all of us to put our hobbies and other commitments on hold during this time. They wanted us to put all our focus and best effort into the prac. Even so, we knew we'd keep dancing during this time; we always dance, no matter what else is happening in our life. In fact, we depend on dance to get us through stressful times. Dancing just feels good. If we have a bad day or something goes wrong, dancing helps us to put that aside and clear our heads. It has always been the thing we turn to; we can't imagine life without it. But we did start to question whether we'd be able to keep making videos for Squared. We knew how long filming and editing took, and we felt that ten videos during our prac would be too much.

We got in touch with Brooklyn and Bailey, and explained our situation. They understood, but they didn't want to see us go because they felt we were doing well on the platform, and they really liked us. They encouraged us to find a solution. None of us was exactly sure how to make it work, but we were open to staying because we were enjoying the experience so much. We'd also been seeing our video views going up each week, which felt pretty good.

Eventually, we decided that the best solution would be to quickly film and edit TEN videos in ONE week! (That's right, one week!) At first, when they suggested we try this, we weren't sure it was even possible. But we discussed it and thought, 'You know what? We can do this.' And somehow . . . we did!

## YouTube famous (at prac)

After that one insane week of filming and editing, we sent all ten videos to Squared and then focused on our last prac. This was kind of a weird time for us, though. We were becoming better known on YouTube, and people were starting to recognise us.

Sometimes, a student would say to one of us, 'We saw you on YouTube last night, Miss!' That would create a strange situation because when we're at school, we're in professional mode; we have different personas at school than in our YouTube videos. It's not that we aren't the same people; it's just that we're there to do a job, and that's teach kids and be someone they can look up to. It's not the place to act fun or silly, like we do in our videos.

Having kids who were familiar with the different side of our life sometimes got awkward. A few of them seemed to think they could take advantage of the fact that they'd seen that other side of us. They'd slack off and think, 'Oh, she's just a fun teacher.' If they tried to get away with stuff, or ask questions related to YouTube, we'd say, 'Thanks so much for watching, but we have to leave this talk outside the school gates.' Eventually, they got the message, and we were able to keep the focus on class, not our YouTube posts!

# Welcome to our channel

By the time we finished uni, we'd been on Squared for a year and had grown a pretty good following. Whenever we signed off for those videos, we'd always say, 'Go and check out our channel,' but even though we did have our own YouTube channel, we never really uploaded videos to it. Occasionally, we'd post little thirty-second montages or short acro videos, but we weren't posting regularly outside of Squared.

We were both offered a teaching job after our pracs (which was a real achievement for us), but we decided to turn them down and dedicate ourselves to our channel for a year. If YouTube went well, we figured we could stay with it and see where it went. If it didn't, we'd become teachers. It was a win-win as far as we were concerned.

In November 2016, we posted our first proper video to our own channel, and we've been posting a video weekly since then. The more time passed, the easier we found it to come up with ideas for content. By the end of that year, we were posting two videos a week: one on our channel and one on Squared. This meant we were much busier filming and editing, but because we were adding to a content schedule we were used to, it wasn't too hard to fit it in.

The idea of working to a theme went out the window after our first six months on Squared. At that point, we were given the freedom to make videos about anything we wanted. Whenever we posted videos of us dancing or doing acro, we noticed that those videos would get more views, so we started getting more creative about how to include those elements in our videos, and how to present things related to acro and dancing. That's what the audience liked, so that's what we wanted to give them.

When it comes to planning content, we are constantly thinking of ideas. If Mum sees something interesting and likes it, she'll tell us. And we each keep lists of video ideas on our phones so we can add to them when inspiration strikes. We also keep a running list of video ideas on a whiteboard at our house. Some of these ideas have been up there for ages. Even though they might not ever happen, we leave them up there because you never know.

With social media, new things come up all the time—trends we want to follow or fun things we want to be a part of. When one of these things comes along, we have a great time thinking about how to add our own spin on it with acro and dance. Often, this fast pace means the idea you'd been planning to film that week gets moved down the list, but that's okay. New things take priority because if you wait too long, the moment passes and you've missed it.

> ### That's the great thing about *working* with *family*: you know they've got your back.

• • •

After we film our videos, we usually split the editing workload; one of us will edit the Squared video, while the other edits the video for our channel. Once we've finished with that, we sit down with Mum to watch the videos. Watching our edits back like this and getting a chance to say, 'I like this' or 'Let's try that', is an important part of our process. After you edit the same footage for hours, you might think it's amazing, but when you show it to someone else, they can see new issues or spot something you haven't noticed.

Very occasionally, we'll disagree about something in a video, but those disagreements are easy to sort out because majority rules. How we deal with things depends on what the issue is and how strongly someone feels about it. If there's something on a video that makes one of us uncomfortable, we'll never go against their wishes. That's the great thing about working with family: you know they've got your back.

Another great thing is that we can be honest and straight up with each other. There's no walking on eggshells. This makes the editing process nice and fast, which is always a good thing!

179

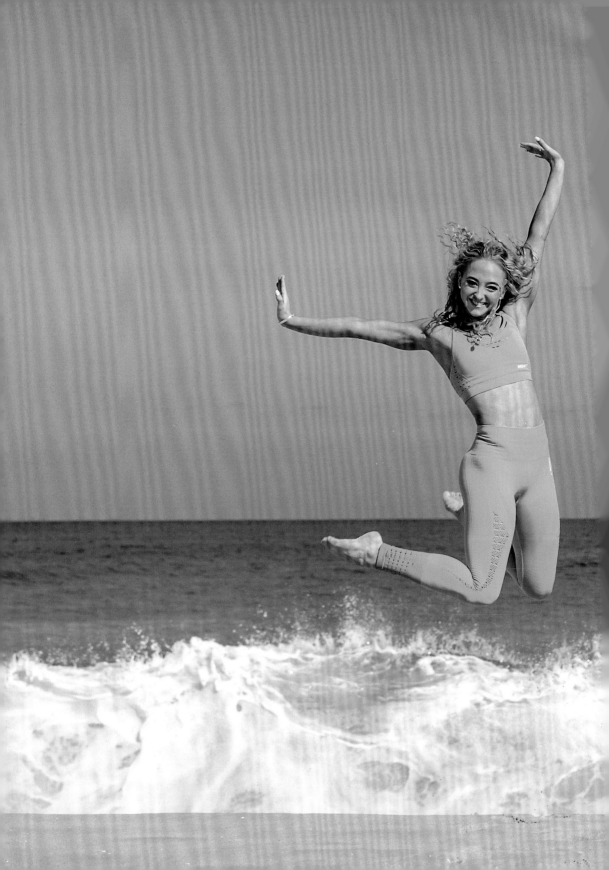

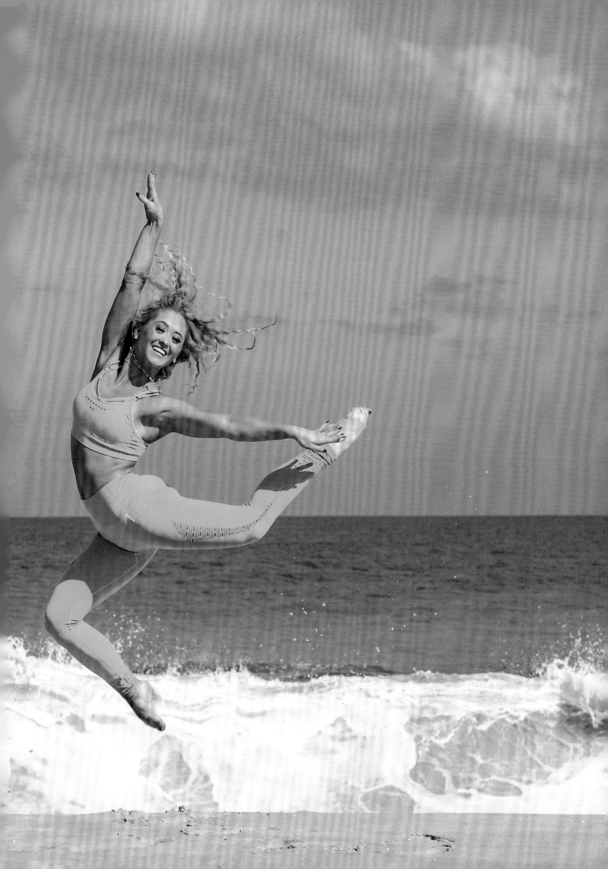

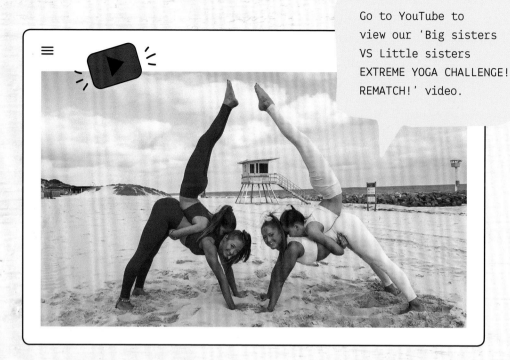

Go to YouTube to view our 'Big sisters VS Little sisters EXTREME YOGA CHALLENGE! REMATCH!' video.

## Our channel goes crazy!

Once we started posting regularly on our own channel, we started growing rapidly. We never expected to grow as fast as we did. The second video we posted on our channel was a yoga challenge, and it went viral in the first week! It ended up getting something like a million views. For one of the videos on our own channel to get those numbers so early on was surprising. The more people that viewed it, the more subscribers we got, so those subscriber numbers shot up, too. It was crazy! It's hard to say why a video goes viral, but looking back at that one, we love the thumbnail for that video: it's vibrant, the beautiful beach is in the background and we're wearing bright colours. Plus, yoga was such a big thing—we must have just caught it at the exact right moment in time.

Can't believe we walked the red carpet with all the stars at the ARIAs in Sydney.

# KEEPING IT REAL

People who share their life on Instagram and social media may look like they have everything together, but no one's life is sunshine and daisies all the time. As great as social media is, it can create a false sense of reality. We often hear people say that Instagram is like a highlight reel of all the best bits in their life— and that's true. The realities of life, like dirty dishes or cleaning your room, aren't as exciting as holiday posts or fashion hauls. The fun and colourful stuff usually makes for better pictures.

It's great to feel motivated or inspired by people you follow and things you see on social media, but you shouldn't ever feel worse about your own life because of what you see there. Always remember that things aren't what they seem behind the scenes—you never know what's going on behind that camera. As long as you're out there every day trying to live your best real life, it doesn't matter what anyone else is doing or posting.

183

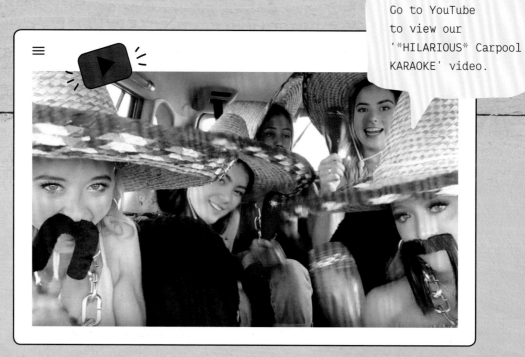

Go to YouTube to view our '*HILARIOUS* Carpool KARAOKE' video.

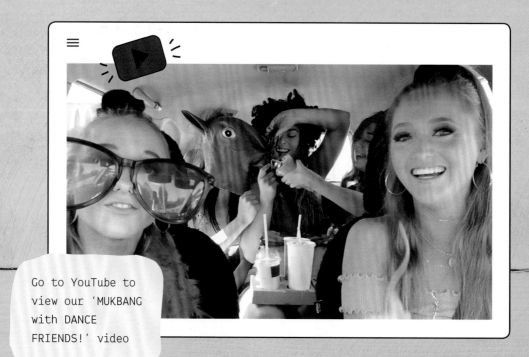

Go to YouTube to view our 'MUKBANG with DANCE FRIENDS!' video

TWINNING IT!

That's the thing with YouTube: you never know with why some videos hit and some don't. You create each video with the same amount of attention, and put a lot of thought, hard work and energy into making each one, and then you hope that it does well. If it works, you think, was the title really good? Did the thumbnail pull them in? Did YouTube push this video out there more than others? You just don't know. Nobody does! You're either lucky or you're not.

Sometimes we'll put out a video and feel confident about it, but it won't go well and we don't know why. It's very up and down—never predictable. There are truly wonderful things about being a YouTuber, but there's no denying that you're on edge all the time because you're always wondering, is this going to perform as well as last week? Are people going to keep watching? It's only natural to take it a bit personally when the views aren't that great. We can't control any of that, though, so we try not to let it distract us. We keep each other upbeat and remind each other that we have to move on and look forward to the next thing. In the end, we just keep doing our best and hope that people like it!

A car karaoke video we did not that long ago is a perfect example of us putting a lot of effort into something that didn't get a lot of views. We were so excited about doing this video (well, two videos, because we split it into two parts). We got a few of our good friends to be in the video with us, and we went out and bought props and outfits for all of us to wear while we danced and did karaoke in our car. Getting the music, outfits and choreography together for that video was a lot of work! And although we had so much fun and love how those videos turned out, they didn't do quite as well as we'd expected. We were a bit disappointed. But after we finished filming, one of our friends said, 'I haven't had this much fun since I was little!' And that was an awesome feeling. It helped remind us of how lucky we are, even when things don't go perfectly.

If you see YouTube in your future, one of the main things we'd say to you is don't get disheartened. If something doesn't go well straight away, hang in there. Staying positive and not giving up is a big part of success, because it's so normal to have a good week sometimes and then a not-so-good week the next. Make the decision to stay committed for whatever period of time feels right for you. Even if we have the worst week of our lives, we always post a video because that's the commitment we've made to ourselves and our subscribers.

Naturally, life gets in the way sometimes. That's normal. But when it does, we go with it and do the best we can. We've definitely had weeks where we've needed to film videos even though one of us has lost their voice or has been sick. Even the week Dad passed away, we still posted a video. We'd already filmed it a few days before, but we also filmed one for the next week, too. Thinking back, we probably needed to distract ourselves from what was going on. Somehow, we pulled ourselves together and just did it. When it comes down to it, we are so grateful for our followers. They give us so much support, in ways they probably don't even realise.

## A million subscribers!

Before that first full year of dedicating ourselves to our own YouTube channel was up, we hit one million subscribers—on 26 September 2017 to be exact! That felt like the most amazing thing in the world to us; we really couldn't believe it. After that viral video, we'd been lucky enough to hit 100,000 subscribers pretty quickly. When that happens, you get a silver play button as a gift from YouTube. It's a representation of all the hard work, so it was nice to get.

After that, the next milestone is 200,000, but we just couldn't wait to hit that one million mark and get another play button trophy from YouTube. Striving for that goal became the next thing for us to work towards.

As our subscriber numbers ticked up, we started watching closely because we wanted to throw a party and film the moment when it happened. But we soon realised it was going to be too hard to capture; sometimes the numbers go up a lot overnight, so it's hard to predict exactly when you're going to hit a particular milestone.

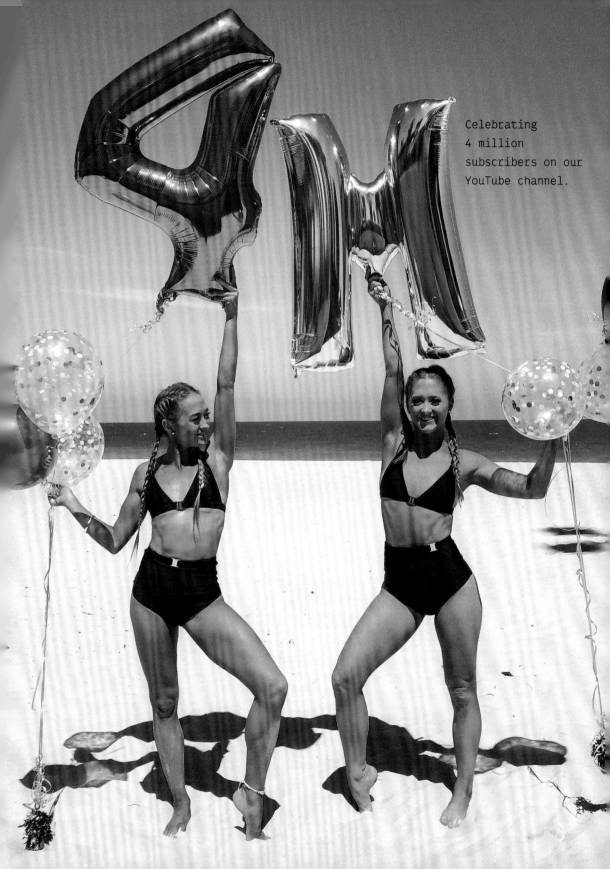

Celebrating
4 million
subscribers on our
YouTube channel.

Instead, we decided to make a montage of us gearing up until we hit the million mark.

It's easy to hop on and off social media all day long, especially when it's also what you do for a job! But as much as we both love our scrolling time, we also like to have plenty of time away from it. It's important not to get too caught up in that online world. We need time away to do all the other things we love in life, like spending time with our family and friends.

When it comes to our YouTube numbers, Mum is really good at keeping us up to date with the statistics. This is nice for us, because it means we don't feel we have to look at that all the time.

Whenever we post a video, we'll stay online for the first hour or so after it goes up. We love being online during this time so we can interact with anyone watching. We'll read the comments, heart them and reply to people. It's great to hear feedback on the video and have that connection with the people who come back week after week. After that first hour, we'll check in randomly when we have time. We honestly have the best followers, and we're so grateful.

We'd love to do a meet and greet so we can meet some of our followers. We talk about this—how exciting it's going to be to meet all the people who have supported us on YouTube and Instagram. It's one of the ways we'd love to give back and say thank you—we know how exciting it is to meet someone you follow. (This book you're reading is another way for us to do that. Hopefully, you're loving it!)

Owning our own business was never the goal when we started out. When we received our first payment from YouTube, we already loved making videos and were planning to continue regardless of whether or not we made money. So, to get paid for it was incredible. That was the moment that opened our minds to bigger possibilities. We suddenly realised, 'Wow, this could be our full-time job if we keep at it and stay focused.'

People might see our videos online and think it's easy to be a YouTuber, but just like any job, there's hard work behind the sunshine and smiles, as well as plenty of ups and downs. You can plan all you like, but problems are bound to come up. You might show up to a location to find there's no extension cord, a background isn't what you expected, or the weather is terrible. Everything takes much longer than we imagine. But we still love doing it!

If you're thinking about trying YouTube, finding what works for you is the key. You need to have a passion and truly love whatever it is you are sharing. When you enjoy what you are doing, it shines through in your videos, and people will find you. But in saying that, in addition to working hard and staying consistent, you also have to be lucky and get a break, because everyone on YouTube wants to be successful. There's so much competition; movie and TV stars even have their own channels now.

When you *enjoy* what you are doing it *shines* through in your videos and people will find you ... but you also have to be *lucky.*

• • •

Despite all the competition, we still think it's an exciting world to be part of. Not long ago, if you wanted to find an audience to share your passion with, you had to audition for panels of casting agents or impress certain people. And if those people didn't value what you were sharing, then too bad! Now, you can make videos from your backyard and let the audience make up its own mind. And that's an amazing thing. Imagine how many entertaining people the world would be missing out on if YouTube didn't exist!

There's a whole world of viewers out there, and so many niches and interests that can capture a passionate audience. Who's to say that your video won't be the thing that lots of people get excited about? If you have a dream, go for it.

189

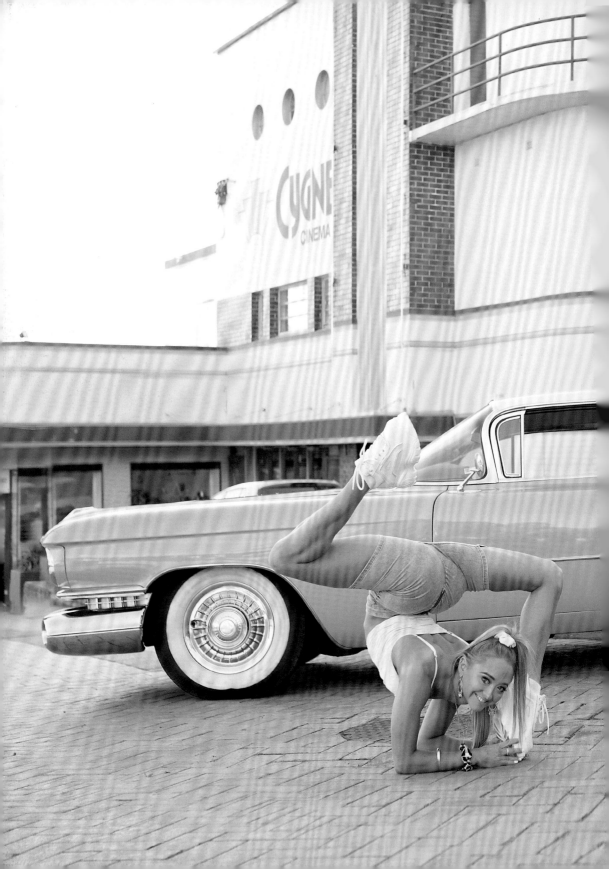

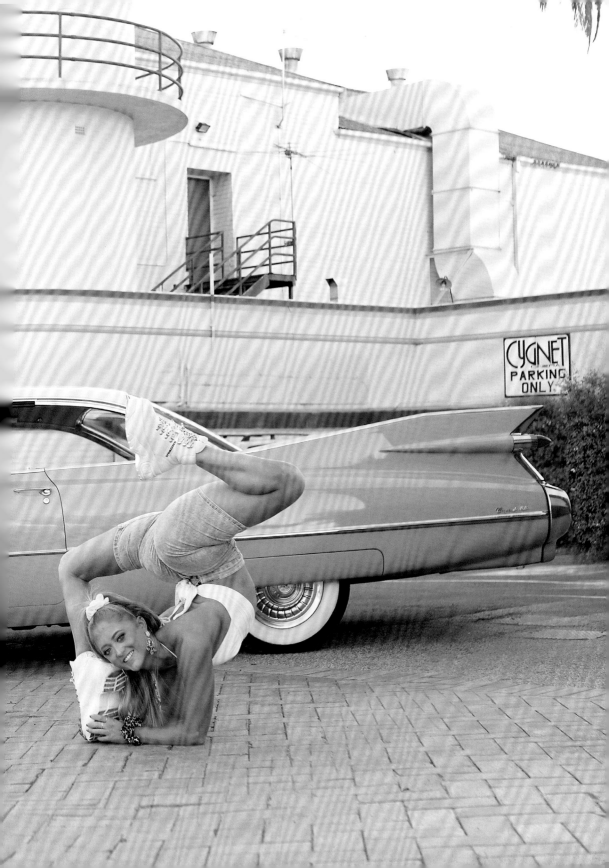

## CHAPTER 9

# Chase your dreams

**D**ancing has brought us everything in life: passion, excitement, opportunity, friends, travel, careers, our amazing online communities . . . even this book!

We hope that you've enjoyed sharing our stories. If you have something in your life that you love doing, we hope you feel inspired to stick with it and keep working hard, even if you aren't sure where it will lead. And if you haven't found your 'thing' yet, hopefully you feel motivated to try some new activities and discover where your talents and passions lie. Everyone has their own special talents!

So many of our dreams have already come true. When we look at what we've crossed off our list in the past few years, we have to pinch ourselves! It's too unreal. This has taught us that we can dream even bigger.

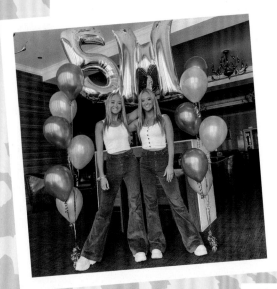

5 Million subs ...
WHAT??? Thank you
so much for your
incredible support.
We love you all!

# Goals we've crossed off

~~Perform on national TV~~

~~Graduate from university~~

~~Complete and pass final CSTD ballet exam~~

~~Meet and perform for Dance Moms star Abby Lee Miller and the girls~~

~~Meet Katy Perry~~

~~Reach 1 million subscribers on YouTube~~

~~Verified on Instagram~~

# You've got to see it to believe it

Some people believe that if you visualise what you want in your mind and believe that it's real, you can make it real in your life. (One of our brothers used to sleep with a $100 note stuck on the ceiling above his bed because he wanted to be a millionaire!)

We figured, why not try it? You never know what the next month or even year will bring. These are the goals we're reaching for now . . .

- 🤍 Create our very own Rybka Twins clothing and activewear range
- 🤍 Perform on *Ellen* (we love her and her show!)
- 🤍 Feature in a pop star's official music video
- 🤍 Be the live act on stage for a pop star, maybe when they're offstage getting changed
- 🤍 Keep growing and evolving on YouTube
- 🤍 Perform at an awards night, like the GRAMMYs
- 🤍 Appear in a movie

And finally, the biggest goal of all: We want to tour so we can say hi to all of you!

We wouldn't be where we are without you, and we are so appreciative. We are just like any normal kids from any normal suburb, and any of you could be where we are today with hard work, determination, passion and a little luck.

Reach for your dreams!

Dream Big

You never know what the future will bring.

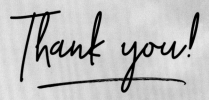

# Thank you!

We'd like to sincerely acknowledge all the people who have helped us on this journey of writing and publishing this book!

To the woman behind the camera and our biggest inspiration and supporter, our mum. It's hard to put into words how truly thankful we are for everything she's done and continues to do for us. Everything we are, she's helped us to be! She's been there from the very beginning and we feel so lucky to have such a caring and loving mum who only ever wants the best for us! We make such a great team and we only ever want to make her proud. We love you so much Mum! THANK YOU! xo

Our family, you mean the world to us and we love you all very much! Thank you for being there and supporting us from the beginning!

Our friends near and far . . . Thank you for bringing out the best in us and for the incredible memories we've made and the adventures we've had together. Each of you has a special place in our hearts. We can't wait to make more memories with you all.

Our past and present dance teachers, thank you for helping to shape us into the dancers we are today. We couldn't have done it without your love, guidance and expertise.

Our talented photographers, Cathy Britton and Yussy Arkam, thank you so much for taking the time to take such beautiful photos for our book. The photos speak for themselves! We will be forever grateful for your ability to capture the moment and bring our visions to life.

A book is a big task that requires an amazing writing and publishing team, which we were lucky to have.

And finally, but definitely not least, thank you from the bottom of our hearts to each and every single one of you for reading this book. (Well done for making it all the way to the end!) Your constant love and the support you show us is inspiring. Thank you for giving us a voice, and the opportunity to share our passion and love for what we do with all of you.

*Teagan xo*

*Sam xo*

Published in 2019 by Murdoch Books, an imprint of Allen & Unwin

Murdoch Books Australia
83 Alexander Street,
Crows Nest NSW 2065
Phone: +61 (0)2 8425 0100
murdochbooks.com.au
info@murdochbooks.com.au

Murdoch Books UK
Ormond House, 26–27 Boswell Street,
London WC1N 3JZ
Phone: +44 (0) 20 8785 5995
murdochbooks.co.uk
info@murdochbooks.co.uk

For corporate orders and custom publishing, contact our business development team at
salesenquiries@murdochbooks.com.au

Publisher: Kelly Doust
Creative Direction: northwoodgreen.com
Editorial Manager: Julie Mazur Tribe
Editor: Kylie Walker
Production Director: Lou Playfair
Photographers: Cathy Britton (pages 2, 4–5, 25, 40–1, 43, 49, 58–9, 76–7, 93, 109, 110–11, 149, 169, 180–1, 190–1) and Yussy Arkam (pages 21, 36, 88–9, 101, 120, 126–7)

Text © Sam Rybka and Teagan Rybka 2019
Text: Sam Rybka and Teagan Rybka with Katie Bosher
Photography © Sam Rybka and Teagan Rybka 2019
Design © Murdoch Books 2019
Cover photography by Cathy Britton, except image on back cover (bottom) by Yussy Arkam

ISBN 978 1 76052 493 7 Australia
ISBN 978 1 91163 240 5 UK

A cataloguing-in-publication entry is available from the catalogue of the National Library of Australia at nla.gov.au
A catalogue record for this book is available from the British Library

Colour reproduction by Splitting Image Colour Studio Pty Ltd, Clayton, Victoria
Printed by C & C Offset Printing Co. Ltd., China

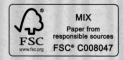

MIX
Paper from
responsible sources
FSC® C008047

The paper in this book is FSC® certified.
FSC® promotes environmentally responsible,
socially beneficial and economically viable
management of the world's forests.